a LANGE medical book

# CURRENT ESSENTIALS: NEPHROLOGY & HYPERTENSION

**Edited by**

**Edgar V. Lerma, MD**
*Clinical Associate Professor of Medicine*
*Section of Nephrology*
*Department of Internal Medicine*
*University of Illinois at Chicago College of Medicine*
*Associates in Nephrology, SC*
*Chicago, Illinois*

**Jeffrey S. Berns, MD**
*Professor of Medicine and Pediatrics*
*Associate Dean for Graduate Medical Education*
*The Perelman School of Medicine at the University of Pennsylvania*
*Philadelphia, Pennsylvania*

**Allen R. Nissenson, MD**
*Emeritus Professor of Medicine*
*David Geffen School of Medicine at UCLA*
*Los Angeles, California*
*Chief Medical Officer*
*DaVita Inc.*
*El Segundo, California*

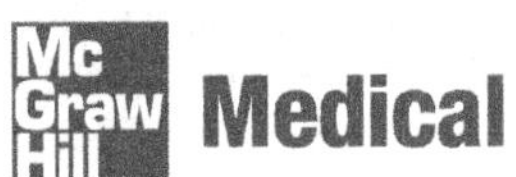

New York   Chicago   San Francisco   Lisbon   London   Madrid   Mexico City
Milan   New Delhi   San Juan   Seoul   Singapore   Sydney   Toronto

**Current Essentials: Nephrology & Hypertension**



1 2 3 4 5 6 7 8 9 0    DOC/DOC    17 16 15 14 13 12

ISBN 978-0-07-144903-8
MHID 0-07-144903-5
ISSN 2166-0387

---

### NOTICE

Medicine is an ever-changing science. As new research and clinical experience broaden our knowledge, changes in treatment and drug therapy are required. The authors and the publisher of this work have checked with sources believed to be reliable in their efforts to provide information that is complete and generally in accord with the standards accepted at the time of publication. However, in view of the possibility of human error or changes in medical sciences, neither the authors nor the publisher nor any other party who has been involved in the preparation or publication of this work warrants that the information contained herein is in every respect accurate or complete, and they disclaim all responsibility for any errors or omissions or for the results obtained from use of the information contained in this work. Readers are encouraged to confirm the information contained herein with other sources. For example and in particular, readers are advised to check the product information sheet included in the package of each drug they plan to administer to be certain that the information contained in this work is accurate and that changes have not been made in the recommended dose or in the contraindications for administration. This recommendation is of particular importance in connection with new or infrequently used drugs.

---

This book was set in Times Roman by Cenveo Publisher Services.
The editors were Christine Dietrich and Harriet Lebowitz.
The production supervisor was Catherine Saggese.
RR Donnelly was printer and binder.
This book is printed on acid-free paper.

International Edition ISBN 978-0-07-128738-8, MHID 0-07-128738-8.
Copyright © 2012. Exclusive rights by The McGraw-Hill Companies, Inc., for manufacture and export. This book cannot be re-exported from the country to which it is consigned by McGraw-Hill. The International Edition is not available in North America.

# Contents

# Contributors

**Jasvinder S. Bhatia, MD**
Boston University School of Medicine
Boston, Massachusetts

**C. Michael Chaknos, MD**
The Perelman School of Medicine
University of Pennsylvania
Philadelphia, Pennsylvania

**Joline Chen, MD**
Boston University School of Medicine
Boston, Massachusetts

**Bhavna Chopra, MD**
The Perelman School of Medicine
University of Pennsylvania
Philadelphia, Pennsylvania

**Richard Glassock, MD**
David Geffen School of Medicine
Los Angeles, California

**Danny Haddad, MD**
The Perelman School of Medicine
University of Pennsylvania
Philadelphia, Pennsylvania

**Ramy Hanna, MD**
David Geffen School of Medicine
UCLA Olive View Medical Center
Los Angeles, California

**Jonathan Hogan, MD**
The Perelman School of Medicine
University of Pennsylvania
Philadelphia, Pennsylvania

**Dany Issa, MD**
The Perelman School of Medicine
University of Pennsylvania
Philadelphia, Pennsylvania

**Mohammad Kamgar, MD**
David Geffen School of Medicine
Ronald Reagan UCLA Medical Center
Los Angeles, California

**Reza Khorsan, MD**
David Geffen School of Medicine
UCLA Olive View Medical Center
Los Angeles, California

**Farrukh Koraishy, MD**
Yale University School of Medicine
New Haven, Connecticut

**Joseph Kupferman, MD**
The Perelman School of Medicine
University of Pennsylvania
Philadelphia, Pennsylvania

**Christine Lau, MD**
David Geffen School of Medicine
Ronald Reagan UCLA Medical Center
Los Angeles, California

**Veena Manjunath, MD**
Yale University School of Medicine
New Haven, Connecticut

**Laura Mariani, MD**
The Perelman School of Medicine
University of Pennsylvania
Philadelphia, Pennsylvania

**Hashim Mohmand, MD**
The Perelman School of Medicine
University of Pennsylvania
Philadelphia, Pennsylvania

**Jacquelyn Nguyen, MD**
David Geffen School of Medicine
UCLA Olive View Medical Center
Los Angeles, California

**Niloofar Nobakht, MD**
David Geffen School of Medicine
Ronald Reagan UCLA Medical Center
Los Angeles, California

**Sefali Parikh, MD**
David Geffen School of Medicine
Ronald Reagan UCLA Medical Center
Los Angeles, California

**Mark A. Perazella, MD**
Yale University School of Medicine
New Haven, Connecticut

**Anjay Rastogi, MD, PhD**
David Geffen School of Medicine
Ronald Reagan UCLA Medical Center
Los Angeles, California

**James Reilly, MD**
The Perelman School of Medicine
University of Pennsylvania
Philadelphia, Pennsylvania

**Earl Rudolph, DO**
Georgetown University
Washington DC

**David J. Salant, MB, BCh**
Boston University School of Medicine
Boston, Massachusetts

**Adam M. Segal, MB, BCh**
Boston University School of Medicine
Boston, Massachusetts

**Swathi Singanamala, MD**
Yale University School of Medicine
New Haven, Connecticut

**Karandeep Singh, MD**
David Geffen School of Medicine
Ronald Reagan UCLA Medical Center
Los Angeles, California

**Christine Vigneault, MD**
Yale University School of Medicine
New Haven, Connecticut

**F. Perry Wilson, MD**
The Perelman School of Medicine
University of Pennsylvania
Philadelphia, Pennsylvania

**Xiaoyi Ye, MD**
David Geffen School of Medicine
Ronald Reagan UCLA Medical Center
Los Angeles, California

# Preface

We are pleased to present this book as a companion handbook to the first edition of *Current Diagnosis and Treatment: Nephrology & Hypertension*. Our goal was to create a quick reference to common presentations of various diseases affecting the kidneys in order to assist clinicians and trainees in providing expert care for their patients with kidney diseases, hypertension, and kidney transplantation. The book follows the *Current Essentials* series format providing a page for each diagnosis with bullet points underneath three headings: Essentials of Diagnosis, Differential Diagnosis, and Treatment. In addition, included in almost all topics is a Pearl and a reference. The book is organized into sixteen sections and six subsections.

We are grateful to the section contributors for their commitment to help us create this first edition. In addition we would like to acknowledge James Shanahan and Harriet Lebowitz and their outstanding team at McGraw-Hill that provided expert guidance and support throughout the project. Lastly, we would like to acknowledge the patience, love, and support of our families for all of our endeavors and in particular for their understanding of the time needed away from them to complete this book.

Edgar V. Lerma, MD
Jeffrey S. Berns, MD
Allen R. Nissenson, MD

# 1

# Fluids & Electrolytes, & Acid-Base Disorders

# 1.1

# Disorders of Volume Regulation

## Diuretic Abuse

- ■ **Essentials of Diagnosis.**
    - Commonly noted in patients who would like to lose weight, especially in females. A variety of complications with electrolyte balance can be noted with surreptitious use of diuretics.
    - Hypokalemic metabolic alkalosis with volume depletion, associated with increased urinary sodium and chloride concentration (Bulimia causes low urinary chloride concentration).
    - Diuretic screen in the urine.

- ■ **Differential Diagnosis**
    - Inherited renal salt wasting disorders (Bartter, Gitelman syndrome).

- ■ **Treatment**
    - Discontinue use of diuretics; use only when indicated.

- ■ **Pearl**

*Consider diuretic abuse in patients with otherwise unexplained hypokalemia and metabolic alkalosis.*

Reference
Greenberg A: Diuretic complications. Am J Med Sci 2000;319:10.

## Diuretic Resistance

- **Essentials of Diagnosis**
  - Inadequate reduction in ECF volume despite near maximal doses of loop diuretics (generally intravenously).
  - Causes include worsening of CHF or cirrhosis, chronic kidney disease, impaired delivery of diuretic to active site in the kidney, chronic diuretic use with intrarenal adaptations limiting diuretic response, and interfering medications (such as NSAIDs) which inhibit secretion of diuretics into the tubules.

- **Treatment**
  - Intravenous diuretics: If patient has been receiving only oral diuretics, a trial of IV diuretics in adequate doses (ie, furosemide up to 80–120 mg IV or equivalent dose of other loop diuretic) is often helpful.
  - Combination diuretic therapy: Combine loop diuretic with thiazide or thiazide-like diuretic (active in distal convoluted tubule), acetazolamide (active mostly in proximal tubule; used to treat or prevent metabolic alkalosis), spironolactone or eplerenone (active in distal tubule; used in patients with cirrhosis, hypokalemia). Patients need to be carefully watched for ECF volume depletion, electrolyte abnormalities (hypokalemia, hypo- or hypernatremia).
  - Continuous diuretic infusion: Avoids peaks and troughs of bolus administration and salt retention after diuretic effect wears off; dose can be easily titrated in intensive care setting.
  - Ultrafiltration: If diuretic therapy fails and the patient is still volume overloaded, ultrafiltration with hemodialysis, peritoneal dialysis, or continuous renal replacement therapy can be used for volume removal depending on indications, blood pressure, and urgency of volume removal.

- **Pearl**

*In patients with diuretic resistance consider and investigate for nephrotic syndrome, nonadherence, use of NSAIDs, and excessive dietary salt intake.*

Reference

Ellison DH: Diuretic resistance: physiology and therapeutics. Semin Nephrol 1999;19:581.

## Edema

- **Essentials of Diagnosis**
  - Edema is palpable swelling caused by increased interstitial fluid volume. Massive accumulation of fluid in the interstitium is called *anasarca*, often associated with both edema and ascites.
  - Mechanisms of formation include:
    - Increased renal sodium retention (CHF, cirrhosis, acute and chronic kidney disease, nephrotic syndrome), pregnancy.
    - Hypoalbuminemia with decreased oncotic pressure (nephrotic syndrome, protein-losing enteropathy, cirrhosis, malnutrition).
    - Venous or lymphatic obstruction.
    - Increased capillary permeability (burns, trauma, sepsis, allergic reaction, some medications such as dihydropyridine calcium channel blockers).
    - Hypothyroidism (pretibial myxedema).
    - Idiopathic edema, cyclic edema.
    - Capillary leak syndrome.
    - Diuretic induced edema (rarely occurs when diuretics are stopped after chronic use).
    - Refeeding; or binging after a period of fasting.

- **Treatment**
  - Treat underlying disorder.
  - Restriction of dietary sodium intake.
  - Diuretics: the diuretic of choice may vary in certain conditions.
    - Cirrhosis: loop diuretic with aldosterone antagonist.
    - CHF and kidney disease: loop diuretics, if necessary with thiazide diuretic.
  - Elevation of extremities for dependent edema, edema related to venous or lymphatic obstruction.
  - Pressure stockings.

- **Pearl**

*In hospitalized patients examine dependent areas such as posterior thighs, back, and sacral area because edema in the lower extremities may not be apparent, leading to the erroneous conclusion that edema has resolved if only the lower extremities are examined.*

Reference

Schrier RW et al: Pathogenesis and management of sodium and water retention in cardiac failure and cirrhosis. Semin Nephrol 2001;21:157.

## Extracellular Fluid Volume Depletion

### ■ Essentials of Diagnosis

- Extracellular fluid (ECF) volume depletion occurs when loss of sodium and water from the ECF exceeds intake.
- Gastrointestinal losses: vomiting, diarrhea, external drainage; Renal losses: diuretics, solute diuresis, mineralocorticoid deficiency; Cutaneous losses: sweat and burns; Third space sequestration: intestinal obstruction, acute pancreatitis.
- Symptoms and signs include: fatigue, thirst, muscle cramps, dizziness, confusion, orthostatic hypotension, decreased jugular venous pressure, hypotension, dry mucous membranes, decreased skin turgor, decreased urine volume.
- Laboratory abnormalities include:
  - Low urine sodium (Na) concentration (<20 mEq/L) and fractional excretion of sodium (FENa) not affected by urine volume (<3%).
  - High urine osmolarity and specific gravity.
  - Elevated BUN:serum creatinine ratio (>20).
  - May be hyponatremia, hypernatremia, or normal serum sodium concentration.
  - Often with evidence of "hemoconcentration": elevated hematocrit, hemoglobin, albumin.

### ■ Treatment

Fluid resuscitation should be done early to prevent systemic hypoperfusion and end-organ tissue injury. Intravenous istotonic saline (0.9% sodium chloride) or lactated Ringer's solution are most commonly used to restore ECF volume initially and should be given at a rate determined by severity of ECF volume depletion (ie, more rapidly if hypotension is present) with monitoring of vital signs and urine output. Other electrolytes should be replaced as indicated. If hypo- or hypernatremic, other IV solutions may need to be given but volume depletion should be at least partially corrected first. Blood transfusion is indicated in cases of hemorrhage.

### ■ Pearl

*Hyponatremia associated with hypovolemia, even if severe, usually corrects with restoration of ECF volume. So hypertonic saline should be avoided, if possible, to avoid overly rapid correction of hyponatremia in such patients.*

Reference

Mehta RL et al: Techniques for assessing and achieving fluid balance in acute renal failure. Curr Opin Crit Care 2002;8:535.

# Renal Salt Wasting Disorders

- ■ **Essentials of Diagnosis**
  - Tubular defect in sodium transport which can result in extracellular fluid (ECF) volume depletion.
  - May occur with or without hyponatremia.
  - Urinary sodium concentration greater than 20 mmol/L.

- ■ **Differential Diagnosis**
  - Chronic kidney disease (CKD), post-ATN or post-obstructive diuresis, adrenal insufficiency, cerebral salt wasting, diuretics, osmotic diuresis (mannitol, urea, glucose), drugs (cis-platinum).
  - Bartter, Gitelman syndromes.
  - Cerebral salt-wasting syndrome.
    - ○ Characterized by hypovolemic hyponatremia secondary to natriuresis; usually seen in patients with CNS disease, particularly subarachnoid hemorrhage.
  - Other laboratory findings: hypokalemia, metabolic alkalosis, elevated BUN, creatinine, and BUN:creatinine ratio, hyponatremia, hypernatremia (with osmotic diuresis, post-ATN or post-obstructive diuresis).

- ■ **Treatment**
  - Replacement of sodium and volume deficit with oral or intravenous sodium chloride; usually with isotonic (0.9% sodium chloride). Hypotonic solutions (ie, 0.45% sodium chloride) may be used in hypernatremic patients if volume deficit is not large. Mineralocorticoid replacement is necessary with adrenal insufficiency.

- ■ **Pearl**

*In patients with relief of long-standing urinary tract obstruction, a useful initial approach is to match urine output exactly with 0.45% saline for the first 24 hours while carefully monitoring vital signs and serum potassium concentration.*

References

Chadha V, Alon US: Hereditary renal tubular disorders. Semin Nephrol 2009;29:399.

Maesaka JK et al: Is it cerebral or renal salt wasting? Kidney Int 2009;76:934.

Singh S et al: Cerebral salt wasting: truths, fallacies, theories, and challenges. Crit Care Med 2002;11:2575.

# 1.2

# Disorders of Water Regulation

## Central Diabetes Insipidus

■ **Essentials of Diagnosis**
  - Deficiency of arginine vasopressin (antidiuretic hormone).
  - Polyuria, polydipsia, mild hypernatremia, elevated serum osmolality (>295 mOsm/kg $H_2O$), and maximally dilute urine (urine <100 mOsm/kg $H_2O$) that resolves with administration of DDAVP or aqueous vasopressin.
  - Can occur in any hypothalamic-pituitary axis disease.
  - CT scan or MRI of hypothalamic/pituitary region may reveal cause.

■ **Differential Diagnosis**
  - Hereditary (rare): both autosomal and dominant forms.
  - Acquired.
    - Head trauma.
    - Pituitary surgery.
    - Neoplasia.
      - Primary: craniopharyngioma, pituitary, suprasellar tumor.
      - Metastatic: leukemia, lymphoma, breast, lung.
    - Vascular.
      - Aneurysm/CVA.
      - Postpartum pituitary necrosis (Sheehan syndrome).
      - Thrombosis.
      - Pregnancy (transient).
    - CNS infection.
      - Any can cause but especially TB and syphilis.
    - Granulomatous disease.
      - Sarcoid, histiocytosis, eosinophilic granuloma.

■ **Treatment**
  - Treat primary process, if possible.
  - Maintain access to free water and encourage patient to drink in response to thirst.
  - DDAVP: desmopressin acetate.
    - Longer duration of action and less vasomotor activity than aqueous vasopressin.
    - Usually intranasal but can be IV or subcutaneous.
    - Dosing interval 8–24 hours as symptoms dictate.

■ **Pearl**
*Patients with central DI with intact thirst and access to free water rarely have significant hypernatremia; treatment with DDAVP or vasopressin aims to reduce inconvenience of polyuria and polydipsia.*

Reference
Adrogue HJ: Hypernatremia. N Engl J Med 2000;342:1493.

# Nephrogenic Diabetes Insipidus

- **Essentials of Diagnosis**
  - Resistance to effect of arginine vasopressin.
  - May have normal or near-normal levels of AVP in serum.
  - Polyuria and polydipsia, hypernatremia (usually mild), elevated serum osmolality (>295 mOsm/kg $H_2O$), and maximally dilute urine (urine <100 mOsm/kg $H_2O$) that does not resolve with administration of DDAVP or vasopressin.

- **Differential Diagnosis**
  - Hereditary.
    - o Mutations in genes for vasopressin (V2) receptor or aquaporin-2 water channel.
    - o Autosomal dominant, recessive, and x-linked described.
  - Acquired (more common).
    - o Chronic kidney disease.
      - Polycystic kidney disease.
      - Obstructive nephropathy.
      - Sickle cell anemia.
    - o Drug-induced.
      - Lithium.
      - Demeclocycline.
      - Amphotericin B.
      - Foscarnet.
    - o Electrolyte disorders.
      - Hypokalemia.
      - Hypercalcemia.

- **Treatment**
  - DDAVP and vasopressin are ineffective.
  - Treat or remove primary cause, if possible.
  - Low-salt diet and thiazide diuretics to induce mild volume depletion and reduce urinary flow.
  - NSAIDS have also been used (reduce GFR).
  - Amiloride can be used in lithium toxicity (blocks collecting duct uptake of lithium ion).

- **Pearl**

*Since patients with nephrogenic DI do not respond to vasopressin, treatment is difficult and patients rely on thirst mechanism and access to water to maintain normal tonicity.*

Reference

Adrogue HJ: Hypernatremia. N Engl J Med 2000;342:1493.

# Hypernatremia with Extracellular Fluid Volume Depletion

## ■ Essentials of Diagnosis
- Occurs when patients sustain losses of both sodium and water with relatively more water loss compared to sodium.
- Total body sodium is decreased with signs of hypovolemia.
- Urine sodium is high (>20 mmol/L) in cases of renal sodium and water loss as opposed to extrarenal losses where urine sodium is less than 20 mmol/L usually.

## ■ Differential Diagnosis
- Use of osmotic or loop diuretics.
- Postobstructive water and sodium losses.
- Excess sweating.
- Burns.
- Diarrhea and other gastrointestinal losses.

## ■ Treatment
- Isotonic saline should be administered to correct the volume deficit.
- Treatment of the cause of hypovolemia and water loss should be pursued.
- Once euvolemia is restored, the water deficit should be calculated and corrected with hypotonic fluids.
- If hypernatremia duration is more that 24 hours, rate of correction of serum sodium should not exceed 1 mEq/L/hour.

## ■ Pearl
*Restore hypovolemia with isotonic fluids with correction of hypernatremia only after correction of ECF volume deficit.*

### Reference
Adrogue HJ, Madias NE: Hypernatremia. N Engl J Med 2000;342:1493.

# Hypernatremia with Extracellular Fluid Volume Expansion

## ■ Essentials of Diagnosis
- Rare, usually iatrogenic form of hypernatremia.
- Serum [$Na^+$] greater than 145 mEq/L with evidence of intravascular volume overload.
- Frequently patients are debilitated (decreased access to free water and/or impaired thirst).
- Gains in total body sodium are greater than gains in total body water.

## ■ Differential Diagnosis
- Hypertonic intravenous fluids (saline or sodium bicarbonate during resuscitation).
- Hypertonic alimentation fluids.
- Dialysis against high sodium dialysate.
- Salt-water drowning.
- Excess mineralocorticoid states (Cushing, primary hyperaldosteronism).
  - o  Clinically significant hypernatremia is quite rare, especially if patients have appropriate water intake.

## ■ Treatment
- Stop offending agents.
- Diuretics (start with loop diuretics).
- Free water repletion may be necessary.
- Consider dialysis in end stage renal disease patients who are hypervolemic.

## ■ Pearl
*Hypervolemic hypernatremia almost always occurs in hospitalized, debilitated patients who receive a sodium load in the setting of impaired thirst and/or inadequate access to free water.*

Reference
Adrogue HJ: Hypernatremia. N Engl J Med 2000;342:1493.

# Hypernatremia with Normal Extracellular Fluid Volume

## ■ Essentials of Diagnosis
- Serum [Na$^+$] greater than 145 mEq/L with euvolemia.
- Loss of total body water without loss of sodium.
- Symptoms: thirst, irritability, lethargy, seizures, coma, and/or death.
- Oliguria and concentrated urine (>700 mOsm/kg $H_2O$).
- Urine [Na$^+$] variable according to sodium intake.

## ■ Differential Diagnosis
- Renal water losses.
  - Diabetes insipidus.
    - Central.
    - Nephrogenic.
  - Normal water excretion with hypodipsia.
    - Impaired thirst.
    - Normal thirst with no access to water.
- Extra-renal water losses.
  - Sweating.
  - Respiratory/mechanical ventilation.
  - Burns.
  - GI losses.

## ■ Treatment
- Estimate free water deficit:
  - $H_2O$ Deficit (L): 0.6 × [Body Wt (kg)] × [([Na$^+$]/140) −1].
- Replacement:
  - Enteral preferred if no contraindications.
  - Can use intravenous 5% Dextrose in water (D5W).
  - Replace over 24–48 hours.
  - Aim for correction of no more than 1–2 mEq/L/hour to avoid cerebral edema.
  - Be sure to replace ongoing losses.
- Treatment directed at primary cause.

## ■ Pearl
*Euvolemic patients with an intact thirst mechanism and access to free water will rarely develop hypernatremia.*

Reference

Adrogue HJ: Hypernatremia. N Engl J Med 2000;342:1493.

# Hyperosmolality

- **Essentials of Diagnosis**
  - Caused by the addition of solute (ie, sodium or glucose) or loss of free water from the extracellular fluid (ECF) space.
  - Loss of free water results in hyperosmolar hypernatremia.
  - Clinical consequences are due to acute shrinkage of cells of the brain as intracellular water moves into the ECF space causing lethargy, weakness, irritability, seizures, and coma.
  - Urea and alcohols (eg, ethanol, methanol, ethylene glycol, isopropyl alcohol) raise ECF osmolarity but are not osmotically active due to equilibration across cell membranes.
  - Compare measured and calculated osmolarity to aid in detection of an exogenous solute; should be within 10 mOsm/L (osmolar gap).

- **Differential Diagnosis**
  - Normal osmolar gap: hypernatremia (due to water loss or sodium ingestion, infusion), hyperglycemia, elevated BUN (azotemia).
  - Elevated osmolal gap.
    - o With elevated anion gap metabolic acidosis: advanced kidney failure, ketoacidosis (diabetic or alcoholic), lactic acidosis (not explained), methanol, ethylene glycol, ethanol (if very severe intoxication).
    - o Without elevated anion gap metabolic acidosis: ethanol ingestion, mannitol, glycine.

- **Treatment**
  - Treat underlying cause using hypotonic intravenous fluids for hyponatremia, insulin for hyperglycemia and diabetic ketoacidosis, dialysis and treatment of poisoning when indicated.

- **Pearl**

*The rate of correction of hypernatremic hyperosmolality should follow the same principles applied for treatment of hyponatremia, so that the serum sodium concentration does not decline faster than 0.5 to 1.0 mEq/L/hour over the first 24 hours.*

References

Hahn RG: Fluid absorption in endoscopic surgery. Br J Anaesth 2006;96:8.

Jammalamadaka D, Raissi S: Ethylene glycol, methanol and isopropyl alcohol intoxication. Am J Med Sci 2010;339:276.

# Hyponatremia

## ■ Essentials of Diagnosis
- Serum [Na$^+$] less than 135 mEq/L resulting from excess of extracellular fluid (ECF) space water relative to sodium.
- May occur with normal, low, or high plasma osmolarity.
- Symptoms, rare if serum sodium concentration is greater than 120 mEq/L unless hyponatremia has developed very rapidly, include headache, lethargy, confusion, ataxia, seizures, coma. Severity of symptoms relate to degree of hyponatremia, rapidity of development, and chronicity. Slowly developing chronic hyponatremia may have few symptoms even if severe.

## ■ Differential Diagnosis
- Pseudohyponatremia: hyponatremia with normal or high plasma osmolarity associated with marked elevations in serum lipids or proteins resulting in artificially low measured serum [Na$^+$] (laboratory artifact).
- Hyperglycemia, mannitol infusion, glycine can cause hyponatremia with normal or high plasma osmolarity due to translocation of water from intracellular to ECF space.
- Hypotonic hyponatremia is due to excess of total body water relative to total body sodium and potassium content. Often related to volume depletion, edematous states, medications (SSRIs, thiazide diuretic, others), SIADH.
- Measure urine sodium, potassium, and osmolarity to calculate free water excretion.
- An important initial step in evaluating hyponatremia is to compare measured and calculated plasma osmolarity.

  Calculated plasma osmolality = 2 × Na (mEq/L) + BUN (mg/dL)/

  2.8 + Glucose (mg/dL)/18

## ■ Treatment
- Hypovolemic hyponatremia: Volume repletion with intravenous isotonic saline (0.9% sodium chloride) or lactated Ringer's solution.
- Euvolemic hyponatremia: Treat underlying diseases (hypothyroidism, adrenal insufficiency), water restriction, stop offending drugs.
- If severe symptoms, treat with hypertonic saline (3% sodium chloride).
- Vaptans, demeclocyline.
- Hypervolemic hyponatremia: treat underlying disorders, often with diuretics, vaptans.
- To minimize the risk of central pontine myelinolysis, the rate of rise in sodium concentration should be no greater than 0.5 to 1.0 mEq/L/hour during the first 24 hours and no more than 18 mEqL in the first 48 hours.

## ■ Pearl
*If hyponatremia develops slowly, symptoms may be absent or mild, and in many patients treatment with fluid restriction, additional sodium intake, and use of loop diuretics will often allow for safe correction without need to use hypertonic saline.*

### Reference
Liamis G et al: Therapeutic approach in patients with dysnatraemias. Nephrol Dial Transplant 2006;21:1564.

# Hyponatremia with Extracellular Fluid Volume Expansion

## ■ Essentials of Diagnosis
- Hyponatremia with low plasma osmolality and elevated urine osmolality (more than 100 mOsm/kg).
- Characterized by low effective circulating arterial volume triggering thirst and antidiuretic hormone release.
- Total body water and total body sodium are increased.
- The patient usually has significant edema.
- Urine sodium is usually low (<20 mmol/L) if renal function is normal.

## ■ Differential Diagnosis
- Congestive heart failure.
- Liver cirrhosis.
- Nephrotic syndrome.

## ■ Treatment
- Manage underlying disease.
- Water and salt restriction.
- Loop diuretics.
- Emerging data suggest a possible role of vaptans in managing hyponatremia in congestive heart failure and liver cirrhosis in selected patients.

## ■ Pearl
*In hypervolemic hyponatremia, the degree of hyponatremia often correlates with the severity and prognosis of the underlying disease, especially in the case of congestive heart failure and liver cirrhosis.*

Reference
Decaux G: Treatment of symptomatic hyponatremia. Am J Med Sci 2003;326:25.

# Hyponatremia with Extracellular Fluid Volume Contraction

## ■ Essentials of Diagnosis
- Hyponatremia with low plasma osmolality and elevated urine osmolality (>100 mOsm/kg).
- Clinical hypovolemia inducing antidiuretic hormone (ADH) release.
- Can be due to renal volume losses (urine sodium >20 mmol/L) or nonrenal losses (urine sodium <20 mmol/L).

## ■ Differential Diagnosis
- Gastrointestinal volume loss including vomiting or diarrhea.
- Third spacing of fluids as in pancreatitis or burns.
- Renal volume losses as in diuretic use and mineralocorticoid deficiency.

## ■ Treatment
- Mainstay of treatment is careful volume expansion to remove the ADH release stimulus.
- Chronic hyponatremia (>48 hours) should be corrected at a rate not exceeding 12 mEq/L in 24 hours to prevent central pontine myelinolysis.

## ■ Pearl
*Hyponatremia due to extracellular volume depletion tends to correct quickly with volume expansion (massive water diuresis), which might require vasopressin or DDAVP and hypotonic fluid administration to slow the rate of correction to a safe range.*

### Reference
Adrogué HJ, Madias NE: Hyponatremia. N Engl J Med 2000;342(21):1581.

# Hyponatremia with Low Plasma Osmolality & Low Urine Osmolality

## ■ Essentials of Diagnosis
- Hyponatremia with low serum osmolality despite a maximally dilute urine and suppressed antidiuretic hormone.
- Urine osmolality usually less than 100 mOsm/kg.
- Usually due to excessive fluid ingestion or inadequate solute intake.
- Large water intake can overwhelm the maximal renal diluting capacity.
- Low solute intake limits the renal ability to excrete water independent of antidiuretic hormone.

## ■ Differential Diagnosis
- Primary polydipsia seen in patients with psychiatric disorders or with lesions affecting the thirst center in the hypothalamus.
- Low solute intake seen in malnourished states like excessive beer drinkers (beer potomania).
- Correction phase of hyponatremia due to other causes.

## ■ Treatment
- Primary polydipsia is treated with water restriction.
- Low-solute-intake hyponatremia is treated by increasing solute intake.

## ■ Pearl
*Unlike patients with hyponatremia due to low solute intake, primary polydipsia patients have a very high urine output (up to 15 L in 24 hours) when they have access to water.*

References

Gillum DM, Linas SL: Water intoxication in a psychotic patient with normal renal water excretion. Am J Med 1984;77(4):773.

Thaler SM et al: "Beer potomania" in non-beer drinkers: effect of low dietary solute intake. Am J Kidney Dis 1998;31(6):1028.

# Hyponatremia with Normal or High Plasma Osmolality

## ■ Essentials of Diagnosis
- Low serum sodium with normal or high plasma tonicity, therefore, not associated with the symptoms of hyponatremia.
- Caused by artifact in measurement of the sodium concentration (pseudohyponatremia) or dilution of serum sodium caused by osmotically active molecules.
- Osmotically active molecules restricted to the extracellular space can draw intracellular water thus diluting the serum sodium concentration without extracellular hypotonicity.
- In pseudohyponatremia, plasma water is overestimated by the clinical laboratory due to the presence of large extracellular molecules, thus reporting a low sodium concentration.

## ■ Differential Diagnosis
- Hyperglycemia in the absence of insulin.
- Mannitol administration.
- Glycine or sorbitol gaining systemic levels, after use in irrigation solutions during hysteroscopy, laparoscopy, or transurethral resection of the prostate.
- Pseudohyponatremia caused by severe hyperproteinemia (like in multiple myeloma) or severe hyperlipidemia.

## ■ Treatment
- No specific treatment as the low plasma osmolality responsible for water shifts in hyponatremia is absent.

## ■ Pearl
*When hyperglycemia is present, the underlying sodium concentration (corrected sodium concentration) can be estimated by adding 1.6–2.4 mEq/L (average of 2 mEq/L) to the reported sodium concentration for every 100 mg/dL increase in plasma glucose above 100 mg/dL.*

References

Hillier TA et al: Hyponatremia: evaluating the correction factor for hyperglycemia. Am J Med 1999;106(4):399.

Weisberg LS: Pseudohyponatremia: a reappraisal. Am J Med 1989;86(3):315.

## Osmotic Diuresis

### ■ Essentials of Diagnosis
- Obligatory urinary water loss due to the presence of a non-reabsorbed solute in the proximal tubule.

### ■ Differential Diagnosis
- Hyperglycemia.
- Mannitol administration.
- High BUN.
- Severe renal failure.
- High protein enteral/parenteral nutrition.
- Catabolic states: burns, critical illness, glucocorticoid administration.
- Urea infusion.
- Hypertonic saline administration.

### ■ Treatment
- Remove offending agents.
- Supportive care.
- Replete water as necessary.

### ■ Pearl
*Hyperglycemia is by far the most common cause of osmotic diuresis.*

Reference

Rose BD, Post TW: Hyperosmolal States-Hypernatremia. In: *Clinical Physiology of Acid-Base and Electrolyte Disorders*, 5th ed. New York, NY: McGraw-Hill; 2001.

## Polyuria

■ **Essentials of Diagnosis**
- Definition: Daily urine output of 3 L or more.
- High serum osmolarity, low urine osmolarity implies diabetes insipidus.
- High serum osmolarity, high urine osmolarity implies osmotic diuresis.
- Low serum osmolarity implies primary polydipsia.
- Obstruction has variable presentations.

■ **Differential Diagnosis**
- Diabetes insipidus (central or nephrogenic).
- Osmotic diuresis.
    - Hyperglycemia.
    - Mannitol administration.
    - High BUN levels.
        - Renal failure.
        - Administration of high protein enteral/parenteral nutrition.
    - Hypertonic saline administration.
- Obstructive diuresis.
    - Occurs during ongoing partial obstruction (eg, prostatic hypertrophy) or after relief of severe obstruction.
    - Usually considered appropriate excretion of overload of solute and water, but can "overshoot" slightly due to mild transient concentrating defect in the collecting ducts.
- Primary polydipsia.

■ **Treatment**
- Discontinue offending osmotic agents, if any.

■ **Pearl**
*Polyuria must be distinguished from urinary frequency, nocturia, dysuria, and incontinence.*

Reference

Rose BD, Post TW: Hyperosmolal States-Hypernatremia. In: *Clinical Physiology of Acid-Base and Electrolyte Disorders,* 5th ed. New York,NY: McGraw-Hill; 2001.

## Syndrome of Inappropriate Antidiuresis

### ■ Essentials of Diagnosis
- Decreased plasma osmolality (<270 mOsm/kg).
- Absence of maximally dilute urinary concentration (>100 mOsm/kg).
- Urine Na concentration greater than 20 mEq/L under normal salt and water intake.
- Absence of adrenal, thyroid, pituitary, or renal insufficiency or diuretic use.
- Low serum uric acid.

### ■ Differential Diagnosis
- Malignancy.
- Pulmonary disease.
- CNS disease.
- Infection.
- Medications associated with hyponatremia.
  - Vasopressin analogues: desmopressin, oxytocin.
  - Drugs that potentiate renal vasopressin: chlorpopamide, cyclophosphamide, NSAIDs.
  - Drugs that enhance vasopressin release: chlorpropamide, clofibrate, carbamazapine, vincristine, nicotine, antipsychotics/antidepressants, ifosfamide, thiazide.

### ■ Treatment
- In the absence of symptoms, conservative approach is appropriate.
- Free water restriction to less than 1 L/day.
- Removal of inciting etiology.
- If euvolemic, saline infusion can worsen the hyponatremia in SIADH.
- If severe impairment in urinary dilutional ability, in case of chronic hyponatremia: V2 receptor antagonists (eg, tolvaptan or conivaptan), demeclocycline.
- For symptomatic chronic euvolemic hyponatremuia, urgent correction with hypertonic saline can be given at 1–2 mL/kg/hour till the serum sodium concentration increases by 2–3 normal/L neurological symptoms resolve and then conservative therapy should be adopted.
- Rate of rise of sodium concentration initially can be about 1mEq/L/hour and should not exceed more than 12 mEq/L/day.
- Low dose loop diuretics have also been used to increase salt and water excretion.

Reference

Ellison DH, Berl T: The syndrome of inappropriate antidiuresis. N Engl J Med 2007;356:2064.

# 1.3

# Disorders of Potassium Metabolism

## Apparent Mineralocorticoid Excess

- **Essentials of Diagnosis**
  - Hypertension with low renin and aldosterone levels.
  - Due to inappropriate action of cortisol on mineralocorticoid receptor.
  - Congenital form: severe hypertension in very young patients caused by 11β-hydroxysteroid dehydrogenase 2 deletion (autosomal recessive inheritance).
  - Adult form: due to overconsumption of licorice (glycyrrhizic acid inhibits 11β-hydroxsteroid dehydrogenase 2).
  - Can also be seen from massive cortisol excess (Cushing syndrome).
  - Hypokalemic alkalosis.
  - Confirm diagnosis by ratio of urinary free cortisol to urinary free cortisone. Ratio greater than 1 is consistent with AME.

- **Differential Diagnosis**
  - Primary hyperaldosteronism.
  - Cushing syndrome.
  - Volume-mediated hypertension.
  - Liddle syndrome.
  - 17-alpha hydroxylase deficiency.
  - 11-beta hydroxylase deficiency.

- **Treatment**
  - Cessation of glycyrrhizic acid consumption.
  - Mineralocorticoid receptor blockade (spironolactone or eplerenone).
  - Dexamethasone may be useful as it suppresses endogenous cortisol without mineralocorticoid effect.

- **Pearl**

*Most licorice in the United States is artificially flavored, but chewing tobacco often contains real licorice.*

Reference

Wilson RC et al: Apparent mineralocorticoid excess. Trends Endocrinol Metab 2001;12:104.

## Bartter Syndrome

- **Essentials of Diagnosis**
  - Genetic defect in the Na/K/2Cl-symporter or other proteins in the thick ascending loope of Henle (usually autosomal recessive).
  - Hypokalemia, metabolic alkalosis, hypotension, and volume depletion.
  - Elevated urinary potassium, chloride, and calcium.
  - Hypereninemic hyperaldosteronism.
  - Neonatal form—severe.
  - Classic form—less severe—presents at 2–3 years of age with polyuria, polydypsia.
  - Kidney stones and nephrocalcinosis in neonatal form.

- **Differential Diagnosis**
  - Loop diuretic abuse.
  - Chronic vomiting (urine chloride levels low).
  - Gitelman syndrome (less severe hypotension, low urinary calcium).

- **Treatment**
  - Liberal sodium and potassium intake.
  - Potassium supplementation.
  - Possibly $K^+$ sparing diuretics.
  - Possibly ACE-inhibition.
  - NSAIDS (neonatal form).

- **Pearl**

*Consider loop diuretic abuse when this syndrome is entertained, especially if diagnosed in an adult.*

Reference

Gill JR: Bartter's syndrome. Annu Rev Med 1980;31:405.

## Gitelman Syndrome

### ■ Essentials of Diagnosis
- Genetic defect in the sodium chloride cotransporter in the distal convoluted tuble (autosomal recessive).
- Hypokalemic metabolic alkalosis.
- Mild volume depletion (patients are often normotensive).
- Elevated urinary chloride, sodium, potassium. Low urinary calcium.

### ■ Differential Diagnosis
- Thiazide diuretic abuse.
- Chronic vomiting (urine chloride levels low, however).
- Bartter syndrome (has more severe volume depletion, high urinary calcium).

### ■ Treatment
- Liberalize sodium intake.
- Potassium supplementation.

### ■ Pearl
*Consider thiazide diuretic abuse when this syndrome is entertained, especially in an adult.*

Reference

Shaer A: Inherited primary renal tubular hypokalemic alkalosis: a review of Gitelman and Bartter syndromes. Am J Med Sci 2001;322:316.

# Gordon Syndrome (pseudohypoaldosteronism)

- **Essentials of Diagnosis**
  - Genetic disorder of *WNK* family kinases (autosomal dominant).
  - Mutation leads to constitutive activation of sodium chloride co-transporter leading to volume expansion.
  - Severe hypertension.
  - Hyperkalemic metabolic acidosis (perhaps, due to decreased distal sodium delivery limiting $K^+$ and $H^+$ exchange or direct effects on ROMK channel from mutation in *WNK*).
  - Hyporeninemic hypoaldosteronism.
  - Short stature, dental anomalies, and intellectual impairment.
  - Improves with thiazide diuretics.

- **Differential Diagnosis**
  - Renal failure with volume expansion.
  - High sodium/potassium intake.

- **Treatment**
  - Thiazide diuretics.
  - Low-salt diet.

- **Pearl**

*Hyperkalemia with normal renal function and hypoaldosteronism should prompt an evaluation for this diagnosis.*

Reference

Gordon RD: Symptom of hypertension and hyperkalemia with normal glomerular filtration rate. Hypertension 1986;8:93.

# Primary Hyperaldosteronism

## ■ Essentials of Diagnosis

- Most common form of secondary hypertension (incidence occurs in 20% of the patients referred for refractory hypertension).
- Hypokalemia and metabolic alkalosis are "classic" but not necessarily present.
- Screening often done with aldosterone to plasma rennin activity ratio more than 30 with elevated plasma aldosterone level and suppressed plasma renin activity.
- Confirm diagnosis with elevated serum aldosterone despite high salt intake.
- High-resolution CT scan or MRI to detect advanced adenomas.
- Bilateral adrenal vein sampling is needed to confirm unilateral versus bilateral diseases.

## ■ Differential Diagnosis

- Adrenal adenoma.
- Glucocorticoid-remediable hyperaldosteronism.
- Gordon syndrome.
- Apparent mineralocorticoid excess.
- Liddle syndrome.
- Esse.

## ■ Treatment

- Surgical excision of adenoma.
- Mineralocorticoid receptor antagonist (spironolactone, epleronone) or amiloride for idiopathic hyperaldosteronism.

## ■ Pearl

*Stop beta blockers, ACE inhibitors, and angiotensin receptor blockers before screening with aldosterone/plasma rennin activity ratio.*

Reference

Ganguly A: Primary aldosteronism. N Engl J Med 1998;339:1828.

## Secondary Hyperaldosteronism

- **Essentials of Diagnosis**
  - High plasma aldosterone levels and volume expansion with hypertension associated with elevated renin.
  - Seen in renal artery stenosis due to renin levels stimulating aldosterone release.
  - Can be seen in severe hypertension with normal renal arteries (presumably due to microvascular damage).
  - Rarely renin-secreting tumors.
  - May be associated with mild hypokalemia and metabolic alkalosis.

- **Differential Diagnosis**
  - Renal artery stenosis.
  - Renin-secreting tumor.
  - Liddle syndrome.
  - Essential (primary) hypertension.
  - Primary hyperaldosteroism.
  - Glucocorticoid-remediable hyperaldosteronism.

- **Treatment**
  - Resection of renin-secreting tumors (often originate within the juxtaglomerular apparatus).
  - Surgery, angioplasty and stenting of renal artery stenosis.
  - Direct renin inhibitors (eg, aliskiren) or K-sparing diuretic.

- **Pearl**

*A high renin and aldosterone may lead to a diagnosis of renal artery stenosis, but intervention in this setting may not improve outcomes.*

Reference

Dworkin LD, Cooper CJ: Clinical practice. Renal-artery stenosis. N Engl J Med 2009;361:1972.

# Hyperkalemia

- **Essentials of Diagnosis**
  - Serum [$K^+$] greater than 5.5 mEq/L.
  - Renal failure (acute and/or chronic) most common cause.
  - Transcellular shift of $K^+$ out of cells into bloodstream.

- **Differential Diagnosis**
  - Renal retention of $K^+$.
    - Acute or chronic renal failure (most common).
    - Renal tubular acidosis (type IV).
    - Aldosterone deficiency or resistance.
    - Drugs: β-blockers, RAAS blockers, NSAIDS, triamterene, amiloride, tacrolimus, cyclosporine, trimethoprim.
  - Extracellular shifts of $K^+$.
    - Insulin deficiency.
    - Hyperosmolar state.
    - Metabolic acidosis.
    - Drugs: succinylcholine, digoxin toxicity, mannitol.
  - Massive release from cells into bloodstream.
    - Rhabdomyolysis, hemolysis, tumor lysis syndrome.
    - Ischemia (especially ischemic gut or hepatic necrosis).
  - Pseudohyperkalemia.

- **Treatment**
  - Identify and reverse cardiotoxicity.
    - EKG shows peaked T-waves early, wide QRS late.
    - Use calcium gluconate or calcium chloride IV (does not remove $K^+$).
    - Anti-arrhythmic effect is immediate, lasts 1–2 hours.
  - Translocate $K^+$ into cells.
    - Insulin infusion (prevent hypoglycemia with glucose).
    - β-agonists (eg, albuterol).
    - $NaHCO_3$ infusion (if patient is acidemic).
  - Increase $K^+$ excretion.
    - Diuretics (loop diuretics first, can add thiazides).
    - Maintain euvolemia to ensure kaliuresis.
    - GI elimination using $K^+$ binding resins.
    - Dialysis in severe or refractory cases.

- **Pearl**

*Identification of the etiology of hyperkalemia must coincide with initial management to guide therapy and reduce recurrence.*

Reference
Nyirenda MJ et al: Hyperkalemia. BMJ 2009;339:b4114.

# Hypoaldosteronism

## ■ Essentials of Diagnosis
- Inappropriate suppression of aldosterone activity.
- Most common presentation in adults is hyperkalemia and metabolic acidosis; hyponatremia can occur.
- Low urine sodium points to primary hypovolemia instead.
- Plasma renin activity, aldosterone, and cortisol levels can be used to differentiate among the three mechanisms.

## ■ Differential Diagnosis
- Decreased activity of the renin-angiotensin system.
  - Hyporeninemic hypoaldosteronism (type IV RTA).
  - Usually with chronic kidney disease (especially diabetics).
  - NSAIDS (by prostaglandin inhibition).
  - ACE inhibitors.
  - HIV/AIDS.
  - Calcineurin inhibitors.
- Decreased aldosterone synthesis.
  - Primary adrenal insufficiency.
  - Aldosterone synthesis intact in secondary/tertiary.
  - Heparin (direct adrenal suppression).
  - Congenital adrenal hyperplasia.
  - 21-Hydroxylase deficiency.
  - Post removal of adrenal adenoma.
- Aldosterone resistance.
  - Angiotensin receptor blockers.
  - Potassium-sparing diuretics.
  - Trimethoprim.
  - Pseudohypoaldosteronism.

## ■ Treatment
- Discontinue offending drugs.
- Fludrocortisone (synthetic mineralocorticoid).
  - Caution in patients with hypertension and/or CKD, as it will induce salt retention.
- Treatment of hyperkalemia.

## ■ Pearl
*If urine sodium is not low, renal function is normal or near-normal, and no obvious cause of hyperkalemia is present, adult patients should be evaluated for hypoaldosteronism.*

Reference
Rose BD, Post TW: Hyperkalemia. In: *Clinical Physiology of Acid-Base and Electrolyte Disorders*, 5th ed. New York, NY: McGraw-Hill; 2001.

# Hypokalemia

## ■ Essentials of Diagnosis
- Serum [K] below 3.5 mEq/L.
- Mild cases asymptomatic.
- Severe hypokalemia can present with flaccid paralysis, respiratory failure, paralytic ileus, and rhabdomyolysis.
- ECG can show prominent U-waves.
- 24-hour urinary [K] excretion (less than 20 mEq) and TTKG (less than 2–3) can help exclude renal [K] wasting.
- Concomitant hypertension, volume expansion, and metabolic alkalosis suggest excessive mineralocorticoid activity.

## ■ Differential Diagnosis
- Most common causes are thiazide or loop diuretics, vomiting/nasogastric suction, and diarrhea.
- Intracellular shift ($\beta$2-agonists, insulin, hypokalemic periodic paralysis).
- Urinary wasting (tubular toxicity from drugs, Liddle syndrome, Bartter syndrome, Gitelman syndrome, bicarbonate-treated type I & II RTA, magnesium deficiency).
- Osmotic diuresis (mannitol, parenteral nutrition, diabetic ketoacidosis).
- Excessive mineralocorticoid activity (primary hyperaldosteronism, Cushing disease, pseudohyperaldosteronism).
- Gastrointestinal losses (ileostomy, ureteral diversion into colon).

## ■ Treatment
- Best treatment is prevention (eg, [K] supplementation with diuretics, using [K]-sparing agents, ACEI, and ARB).
- Oral replacement preferable. KCl for patients with acidosis and K-citrate or K-acetate for those with metabolic acidosis.
- Intravenous replacement can be done via peripheral veins ($\leq$40 mEq/L of fluid) or central veins ($\leq$10–20 mEq/hour).

## ■ Pearl
*In general, plasma [K] between 3 and 3.5 mEq/L represents a K deficit of 200–400 mEq, while a plasma [K] between 2.0 and 3.0 mEq/L requires 400–800 mEq.*

Reference

Gennari FJ: Disorders of potassium homeostasis. Hypokalemia and hyperkalemia. Crit Care Clin 2002;18:273.

# Hypokalemia with High Urinary Potassium Excretion

- ## Essentials of Diagnosis
  - Serum [K] less than 3.5 mEq/L and 24-hour urinary [K] excretion greater than 30 mEq/L (more reliable), spot urinary [K] greater than 20 mEq/L, or transtubular potassium gradient (TTKG) greater than 3.
  - Reflects inappropriate renal loss of potassium either due to intrinsic renal defect or iatrogenic causes.
  - Concomitant hypertension, volume expansion, and metabolic alkalosis suggest excessive mineralocorticoid activity.

- ## Differential Diagnosis
  - Most common causes are thiazide or loop diuretics, vomiting and nasogastric suction.
  - Urinary wasting (tubular toxicity from drugs, Liddle syndrome, Bartter syndrome, Gitelman syndrome, bicarbonate-treated type I & II RTA, magnesium deficiency).
  - Osmotic diuresis (mannitol, parenteral nutrition, diabetic ketoacidosis).
  - Excessive mineralocorticoid activity (primary hyperaldosteronism, Cushing disease, pseudohyperaldosteronism).

- ## Treatment
  - Best treatment is prevention (eg, [K] supplementation with diuretics, using [K]-sparing agents, ACEI, and ARB).
  - Oral replacement is preferable. KCl for patients with alkalosis and K-citrate or K-acetate for those with metabolic acidosis.
  - Intravenous replacement can be done via peripheral veins ($\leq$40 mEq/L of fluid) or central veins ($\leq$10–20 mEq/hour).

- ## Pearl
*Renal wasting can be intermittent (eg, shortly after diuretic administration and during active vomiting and nasogastric suction).*

Reference
Warnock DG: Hereditary disorders of potassium homeostasis. Best Pract Res Clin Endocrinol Metab 2003;17:505.

# Hypokalemia with High Blood Pressure

## ■ Essentials of Diagnosis
- Serum [K] less than 3.5 mEq/L.
- Blood pressure greater than 140/90 mm Hg.
- These conditions are generally characterized by either high aldosterone levels, genetic defects mimicking aldosterone access, or excessive nonaldosterone corticosteroids, either exogenous or endogenous.

## ■ Differential Diagnosis
- Checking plasma renin activity (PRA) and plasma aldosterone concentration (PAC) can help with finding etiology. This can be followed by adrenal vein sampling in some cases to define the laterality.
- High PRA and high PAC: renovascular hypertention, renal infarct, acute glomerulonephritis, diuretics, coarctation of aorta, and renin-secreting tumors.
- Normal to low PRA and high PAC: primary aldosteronism, Conn syndrome (aldosterone-producing adrenal adenoma), bilateral adrenal hyperplasia, glucocorticoid remediable hyperaldosteronism, and aldosterone-producing adrenal carcinoma.
- Low PRA and low PAC: syndrome of apparent mineralocorticoid access, liquorice ingestion, Liddle syndrome, congenital adrenal hyperplasia, exogenous mineralocorticoid, and Cushing syndrome.

## ■ Treatment
- Treat reversible causes.
- Potassium-sparing diuretics are effective in many patients but the choice of diuretic depends upon the specific etiology and patient characteristics.
- Surgical resection of hormone producing tumors may result in cure.
- Oral replacement preferable. KCl for patients with alkalosis and K-citrate or K-acetate for those with metabolic acidosis.
- Intravenous replacement can be done via peripheral veins ($\leq 40$ mEq/L of fluid) or central veins ($\leq 10$–$20$ mEq/hour).

## ■ Pearl
*Adrenal vein sampling can help identify patients with adenoma who may benefit from surgery.*

Reference
Young WF Jr, Hogan MJ: Renin-independent hypermineralocorticoidism. Trends Endocrinol Metab 1994;5:97.

# Hypokalemia with Normal or Low Blood Pressure

## ■ Essentials of Diagnosis
- Serum [K] less than 3.5 mEq/L.
- Blood pressure less than 140/90 mm Hg.
- These conditions are generally characterized by potassium wasting, volume depletion, and secondary hyperaldosteronism.

## ■ Differential Diagnosis
- Diuretics: especially loop and thiazide diuretics.
- Gitelman syndrome: a defect of the thiazide-sensitive NaCl transporter in the early distal renal tubule; characterized by hypocalciuria and severe hypomagnesemia.
- Bartter syndrome: impaired function of the Na-K-2Cl transporter in the thick ascending limb of Henle; characterized by hypercalciuria.
- Osmotic diuresis: hyperglycemia, high blood urea nitrogen (in patients with highly catabolic conditions—like acute illness and high-dose steroids—who are also receiving parenteral nutrition or tube feeding) and mannitol.
- Tubular dysfunction: nephrotoxic drugs (aminoglycoside antibiotics, amphotericin B, cisplatin, and foscarnet) and acute myeloid or lymphoblastic leukemia.
- Poorly reabsorbed nonchloride anion: high-dose Na-penicillin, diabetic ketoacidosis (Na-beta-hydroxybutyrate), inhalation of toluene/glue (Na-hippurate), and during vomiting or nasogastric suction (when sodium bicarbonate spills into the distal tubule and urine).
- Bicarbonate treatment of proximal renal tubular acidosis (RTA type 2).
- Type 1 distal renal tubular acidosis.
- Ureterosigmoidostomy.

## ■ Treatment
- Treat reversible causes.
- Oral replacement preferable. KCl for patients with alkalosis and K-citrate or K-acetate for those with metabolic acidosis.
- Intravenous replacement can be done via peripheral veins ($\leq$ 40 mEq/L of fluid) or central veins ($\leq$10–20 mEq/hour).

## ■ Pearl
*Metabolic acidosis can be seen with acetazolamide, renal tubular acidoses, ureterosigmoidostomy, and glue sniffing.*

Reference

Warnock DG: Hereditary disorders of potassium homeostasis. Best Pract Res Clin Endocrinol Metab 2003;17:505.

# Hypokalemia with Normal or Low Urinary Potassium Excretion

## ■ Essentials of Diagnosis

- Serum [K] less than 3.5 mEq/L and 24-hour urinary [K] excretion less than 30 mEq (more reliable), spot urinary [K] less than 20 mEq/L or transtubular potassium gradient (TTKG) less than 2.
- Reflects extra-renal loss of potassium or shift into intracellular compartment with appropriate renal conservation.
- In cases of potassium shift into intracellular compartment, the urinary potassium excretion can be variable.

## ■ Differential Diagnosis

- Intracellular shift: alkalosis, increase uptake (hyperalimentation, leukemia, insulin), and familial periodic paralysis.
- GI losses: nasogastric suction, diarrhea, villous adenoma, laxative abuse, and ureterosigmoidostomy.
- Skin losses in perspiration.
- Decreased intake: starvation, tea-and-toast diet, and anorexia nervosa.

## ■ Treatment

- Treat or eliminate reversible causes.
- Oral replacement preferable. KCl for patients with alkalosis and K-citrate or K-acetate for those with metabolic acidosis.
- Intravenous replacement can be done via peripheral veins ($\leq$ 40 mEq/L of fluid) or central veins ($\leq$10–20 mEq/hour).

## ■ Pearl

*Concurrent metabolic acidosis generally indicates GI losses.*

### Reference

Gennari FJ: Disorders of potassium homeostasis. Hypokalemia and hyperkalemia. Crit Care Clin 2002;18:273.

# Liddle Syndrome

- **Essentials of Diagnosis**
  - Due to constitutively active epithelial sodium channel (ENaC) in the collecting duct.
  - Autosomal dominant inheritance.
  - Hypokalemic hypertension.
  - Hyporeninemic hypoaldosteronism.
  - Absent response to mineralocorticoid receptor antagonists (aids in differentiating from apparent mineralocorticoid excess).
  - Good response to epithelial sodium channel blockers.

- **Differential Diagnosis**
  - Apparent mineralocorticoid excess.
  - Volume-mediated hypertension.
  - Cushing syndrome.

- **Treatment**
  - Epithelial sodium channel blockers (usually amiloride 5–15 mg twice daily).

- **Pearl**

*Suspect if lack of response to mineralocorticoid receptor antagonists.*

Reference

Hanson JH et al: Hypertension caused by a truncated epithelial sodium channel y subunit: genetic heterogeneity of Liddle syndrome. Nat Gen 1995;11:76.

# Pseudohyperaldosteronism

## ■ Essentials of Diagnosis
- Biochemical and clinical features of mineralocorticoid excess state but with suppressed aldosterone levels.
- Low plasma aldosterone level.
- Low plasma renin activity.
- Serum [K] below 3.5 mEq/L.
- Metabolic alkalosis.
- Hypertension and volume expansion.

## ■ Differential Diagnosis
- Liddle syndrome (gain of function mutation affecting the epithelial sodium channel).
- Secretion of a nonaldosterone mineralocorticoid: deoxycorticosterone-secreting adrenal tumors, some forms of congenital adrenal hyperplasia (17-$\alpha$- and 11-$\beta$-hydroxylase deficiency).
- Syndrome of apparent mineralocorticoid excess (AME): deficiency of the enzyme 11-$\beta$-hydroxysteroid dehydrogenase type 2 (11-$\beta$-HSD2), which inactivates the glucocorticoids, results in abnormal activation of the mineralocorticoid receptor by high levels of cortisol.
- Ingestion of substances containing glycyrrhetinic acid, which antagonizes 11-$\beta$-HSD2 (European licorice, several decongestants available in Europe, and some brands of chewing tobacco.
- Cushing syndrome due to ectopic ACTH secretion (very high levels of cortisol overwhelm 11-$\beta$-HSD2).

## ■ Treatment
- Treat any reversible cause (eg, resection of tumor, stop ingestion of glycyrrhetinic acid containing agent etc).
- Potassium-sparing diuretics (spironolactone, amiloride, and eplerenone) are effective in many types.
- Dexamethasone can be used in AME to decrease the production of cortisol by suppressing ACTH.

## ■ Pearl
*Spironolactone is ineffective in Liddle syndrome as the defect is in the epithelial sodium channel.*

Reference

Warnock DG: Hereditary disorders of potassium homeostasis. Best Pract Res Clin Endocrinol Metab 2003;17:505.

# Pseudohyperkalemia

## ■ Essentials of Diagnosis
- Artifact related to specimen collection or preparation.
- Serum $[K^+]$ exceeds plasma $[K^+]$ by greater than 0.5 mEq/L.

## ■ Differential Diagnosis
- Fist clenching during phlebotomy.
- Prolonged tourniquet application.
- Sample hemolysis (delayed analysis, traumatic venipuncture).
- Extreme leukocytosis ($>100 \times 10^3/\mu L$).
- Extreme thrombocytosis ($>1000 \times 10^3/\mu L$).
- Familial pseudohyperkalemia.
  - Rare, benign, inherited RBC trait predisposing to pseudohyperkalemia if specimen is analyzed hours after collection; fresh samples are unaffected.

## ■ Treatment
- Presume true hyperkalemia and treat until proven otherwise.
- Counsel patient and phlebotomist to avoid common causes.

## ■ Pearl
*Plasma $[K^+]$ is key to diagnosis of pseudohyperkalemia.*

### Reference
Nyirenda MJ et al: Hyperkalaemia. BMJ 2009;339:b4114.

# Pseudohypokalemia

## ■ Essentials of Diagnosis
- Serum [K] below 3.5 mEq/L.
- Can occur if blood specimen from patient with chronic myelocytic leukemia (usually with WBC count $>10^5/\mu L$) remains at room temperature for extended duration before being analyzed (due to uptake of K by abnormal leukocytes). Redrawing a specimen with prompt separation of serum or plasma can confirm diagnosis.
- Seasonal pseudohypokalemia: seen occasionally in specimens collected in outpatient setting in increasing ambient temperature (June to August).

## ■ Differential Diagnosis
- True hypokalemia of any etiology.

## ■ Treatment
- None required.

## ■ Pearl
*Patients will be asymptomatic with normal ECG.*

Reference

Sodi R et al: The phenomenon of seasonal pseudohypokalemia: effects of ambient temperature, plasma glucose and role for sodium-potassium-exchanging-ATPase. Clin Biochem 2009;42(9):813.

# 1.4

# Disorders of Calcium Metabolism

## Hypercalcemia of Malignancy

### ■ Essentials of Diagnosis
- Occurs most commonly in patients with breast or lung cancer, lymphoma, and multiple myeloma.
- Low PTH levels (<25 pg/mL) should be present in the absence of coexistent primary hyperparathyroidism.
- Parathyroid related peptide (PTHrP) level may be elevated.
- Calcitriol levels may be elevated in lymphoma-related hypercalcemia.

### ■ Differential Diagnosis
- Primary hyperparathyroidism, familial hypocalciuric hypercalcemia, granulomatous diseases (ie, sarcoidosis), milk alkali syndrome, thiazide diuretics, immobilization.

### ■ Treatment
- If possible, treat underlying malignancy.
- Avoid calcium supplementation, stop thiazide diuretics.
- Correct any intravascular volume depletion with intravenous isotonic saline.
- Avoid use of loop diuretics in initial therapy unless patient is volume expanded.
- Calcitonin is indicated for acute management given its rapid onset of action.
- IV bisphosphonates have a more delayed onset so are often given initially with expected response to occur after several days.
- Glucocorticoids are often most useful with multiple myeloma and lymphoma.
- Dialysis may be required if hypercalcemia is severe, refractory to treatment, and associated with kidney failure.

### ■ Pearl
*Hypercalcemia of malignancy almost always occurs in patients with known or evident malignancy; the main differential diagnostic issue in asymptomatic patients, and those without a cancer diagnosis, is primary hyperparathyroidism.*

References

Sargent JT, Smith OP: Haematological emergencies managing hypercalcaemia in adults and children with haematological disorders. Br J Haematol 2010;149:465.

Stewart AF: Hypercalcemia associated with cancer. New Engl J Med 2005;352:373.

# Hypercalcemia

## ■ Essentials of Diagnosis
- Clinical manifestations that suggest diagnosis include neuropsychiatric complaints, polyuria, polydipsia, acute kidney injury, nephrolithiasis, and/or constipation.
- Laboratory diagnosis is the mainstay. Always correct for hypoalbuminemia or check ionized calcium.
- PTH will be low in malignancy, sarcoidosis, tuberculosis; PTH will be high in primary hyperparathyroidism.

## ■ Differential Diagnosis
- Malignancy.
- Primary hyperparathyroidism.
- Sarcoidosis.
- Tuberculosis.
- Familial hypocalciuric hypercalcemia (FHH).
- Thiazide diuretics.

## ■ Treatment
- Isotonic saline and/or loop diuretic after volume depletion has been corrected.
- IV calcitonin (acute treatment).
- Bisphosphonates.
- Dialysis.
- Glucocorticoids (for hypercalcemia associated with granulomatous disease).

## ■ Pearl
*The total serum calcium is lower by 0.8 mg/dL (0.2 mmol/L) for every 1.0 g/dL that the serum albumin is below 4 g/dL while the ionized calcium concentration remains normal.*

Reference

Pecherstorfer M et al: Current management strategies for hypercalcemia. Treat Endocrinol 2003;2(4):273.

# Familial Hypocalciuric Hypercalcemia

## ■ Essentials of Diagnosis
- This is an autosomal dominant disorder in which mutation of the *calcium-sensing receptor (CaSR)* gene causes decreased function or lack of function of the CaSR leading to increased renal calcium reabsorption and reduced renal calcium excretion.
- Patients are asymptomatic since symptoms of hypercalcemia are mediated through the CaSR, which is abnormal in this condition.
- Patients present with asymptomatic hypercalcemia, low urinary calcium excretion (<200 mg/24 hour), normal PTH levels (in 80% of cases; PTH level are elevated in about 20% of patients), with high-normal or elevated serum magnesium levels.
- Genetic testing may be indicated in selected patients to distinguish from primary hyperparathyroidism.

## ■ Differential Diagnosis
- Primary hyperparathyroidism.
- Granulomatous disease.
- Thiazide use.

## ■ Treatment
- No treatment is indicated as this is generally an asymptomatic condition.
- Parathyroidectomy is usually not effective and should be avoided.

## ■ Pearl
*Familial hypocalciuric hypercalcemia is a benign, asymptomatic disorder that can be difficult in some patients to distinguish from primary hyperparathyroidism but does not require parathyroidectomy.*

References

Brown EM: Clinical lessons from the calcium-sensing receptor. Nat Clin Pract Endocrinol Metab 2007;3:122.

Riccardi D, Brown EM: Physiology and pathophysiology of the calcium-sensing receptor in the kidney. Am J Physiol Renal Physiol 2010;298:F485.

Varghese J et al: Benign familial hypocalciuric hypercalcemia. Endocr Pract 2011;17(1):13.

# Primary Hyperparathyroidism

## ■ Essentials of Diagnosis
- Usually due to parathyroid adenoma(s).
- Elevated serum and ionized calcium, elevated PTH level, and normal to high levels of urinary calcium.
- Clinical manifestations include nephrolithiasis, chronic kidney disease, neuromuscular symptoms, bone fractures.

## ■ Differential Diagnosis
- Parathyroid adenoma.
- Diffuse parathyroid hyperplasia (limited to end stage renal disease).
- Medications (ie, lithium).
- Multiple endocrine neoplasia (MEN) syndrome.
- Parathyroid carcinoma.

## ■ Treatment
- Surgery for symptomatic disease (kidney stones, renal impairment, bone fractures) or in younger patients.
- Surgery for mild and asymptomatic disease or in older patients.
  - Calcium greater than 1 mg/dL above the upper limit of normal
  - Urinary calcium excretion greater than 400 mg/24 hours
  - Creatinine clearance 30% reduced compared to age-matched healthy patients
  - Bone T-score less than –2.5
  - Age less than 50 years
- Nonsurgical treatment may include the bisphosphonates and calcimimetics (cinacalcet).

## ■ Pearl
*Completely asymptomatic patients with mild hypercalcemia may be observed and treated medically without compromising survival.*

Reference

DeLellis RA et al: Primary hyperparathyroidism: a current perspective. Arch Pathol Lab Med 2008;132(8):1251.

## Secondary Hyperparathyroidism

- **Essentials of Diagnosis**
  - Occurs in advanced kidney disease as a result of decreased 1,25-dihydroxy vitamin D synthesis, hypocalcemia, and phosphate retention.
  - PTH levels can be markedly elevated up to 20–40 times the upper limit of normal.
  - Serum calcium may be low or normal.
  - Can lead to high turnover bone disease and severe skeletal lesions leading to bone pain, deformities, and fractures.

- **Differential Diagnosis**
  - Chronic kidney disease (vast majority).
  - Malabsorption syndromes (eg, pancreatitis, small bowel disease, post-bariatric surgery) as a result of decreased vitamin D absorption in the gut.

- **Treatment**
  - Dietary phosphorus restriction.
  - Active vitamin D analogs (eg, calcitriol, paricalcitol, doxercalciferol).
  - Phosphate binders (both calcium and non-calcium based).
  - Calcimimetics (eg, cinacalet).
  - Surgical—parathyroidectomy.

- **Pearl**

*Untreated secondary hyperparathyroidism can lead to tertiary hyperparathyroidism, where parathyroid hypertrophy and PTH production are irreversible and resistant to biochemical feedback.*

Reference

Eknoyan G et al: Bone metabolism and disease in chronic kidney disease. Am J Kidney Dis 2003;42:1.

## Hypocalcemia

■ **Essentials of Diagnosis**
- Tetany, carpopedal spasms, tingling of lips and hands, muscle and abdominal cramps, psychological changes.
- Positive Chvostek sign and Trousseau sign.
- Can be the result of rapid tissue deposition of calcium or precipitation with other ions such as phosphates.
- Transient hypocalcemia is common in critically ill patients.
- Sustained hypocalcemia can be found in patients with chronic kidney disease secondary to abnormalities in PTH and vitamin D homeostasis.
- Calculate "corrected" calcium concentration with hypoalbuminemia (serum Ca decreases ~ 0.8 mg/dL for each 1 g/dL decrease in serum albumin). Often best to measure ionized calcium directly.

■ **Differential Diagnosis**
- Hypoparathyroidism.
- Post-parathyroidectomy.
- Pseudohypoparathyroidism.
- Advanced chronic kidney disease.
- Chronic hypovitaminosis D.
- Complex formation: pancreatitis, tumor lysis syndrome, rhabdomyolysis, hyperphosphatemia, citrate (blood transfusion).
- Severe hypomagnesemia.

■ **Treatment**
- Treat underlying cause.
- Calcium infusions: calcium gluconate 1–2 g IV over 10–20 min, then 1.0 mg/kg/hr of 10% calcium gluconate if needed.
- Oral calcium supplements, vitamin D supplementation (eg, ergocalciferol, cholecalciferol, calcitriol), correct hypomagnesemia.
- Dialysis in severe renal failure or in setting of tumor lysis syndrome.

■ **Pearl**
*Unless hypocalcemia is symptomatic, avoid intravenous calcium infusion in patients with hypocalcemia and hyperphosphatemia to eliminate risk of soft tissue deposition of calcium-phosphate salts.*

References
Cooper MS, Gittoes NJ: Diagnosis and management of hypocalcaemia. BMJ. 2008;336:1298.
Moe SM: Disorders involving calcium, phosphorus, and magnesium. Prim Care. 2008;35:215.

# Hypoparathyroidism

## ■ Essentials of Diagnosis
- Tetany, carpopedal spasms, tingling of lips and hands, muscle and abdominal cramps, psychological changes.
- Positive Chvostek sign and Trousseau sign.
- Serum calcium low; serum phosphate high; alkaline phosphatase normal; urine calcium excretion reduced.
- Low or low-normal serum PTH in presence of hypocalcemia.
- Serum magnesium may be low.

## ■ Differential Diagnosis
- Acquired: post-surgical, irradiation, heavy metals (copper or iron as in Wilson disease or hemochromatosis).
- Autoimmune: polyglandular autoimmunity (PGA type 1), granulomatous disease, Reidel thyroiditis.
- Congenital forms.
- Other causes of hypocalcemia, including respiratory alkalosis, hypoalbuminemia, malabsorption, medications, etc will be present with similar symptoms and should be considered, but should have normal or elevated PTH.

## ■ Treatment
- IV calcium glunconate: 10–20 mL of 10% solution, given *slowly* until tetany ceases. The rate should be so adjusted so serum calcium is maintained between 8 mg/dL and 9 mg/dL.
- Oral calcium carbonate: 1–3 g daily divided in 2–3 doses.
- Calcitriol: 0.5–2 mcg/d divided into one to two doses daily should be started immediately.
- Ergocalciferol: 25,000–150,000 IU/day, may also be used.
- Target serum calcium (albumin-corrected) should be 8.0–8.5 mg/dL to avoid symptoms of hypocalcemia.

## ■ Pearl
*If hypomagnesemia is present, it must be corrected to treat the resulting hypocalcemia.*

### Reference
Shoback D: Clinical practice. Hypoparathyroidism. N Engl J Med 2008;359(4):391.

## Milk Alkali Syndrome

### ■ Essentials of Diagnosis
- Diagnosis relies on a thorough clinical history for ingestion of calcium-containing compounds.
- Hypercalcemia due to the ingestion of calcium-containing compounds and eventually contributed to by the metabolic alkalosis (decreases calcium excretion) and volume contraction.
- Metabolic alkalosis due to the ingestion of alkali-containing compounds, hypercalcemia, and decreased renal function.
- Renal insufficiency due to hypercalcemia-related renal vasoconstriction.
- Nephrocalcinosis may also occur.
- May present as acute or chronic hypercalcemia.
- PTH and calcitriol levels are usually appropriately low in the setting of hypercalcemia.
- In modern milk alkali syndrome, hypophosphatemia is usually present.

### ■ Differential Diagnosis
- Primary hyperparathyroidism.
- Hypercalcemia of malignancy.
- Familial hypocalciuric hypercalcemia.
- Granulomatous disease.
- Medication induced.
- Immobilization.
- Vitamin D intoxication.

### ■ Treatment
- Discontinue offending agents.
- If severe, treat hypercalcemia and alkalosis with normal saline.
- After volume repletion has occurred, a loop diuretic may be used.
- If severe, may require dialysis.

### ■ Pearl
*The Milk Alkali syndrome is being diagnosed more frequently in the setting of increased use of calcium-containing compounds used for treatment or prevention of osteoporosis.*

Reference
Patel AM, Goldfarb S: Got calcium? Welcome to the calcium-alkali system. J Am Society of Nephrology 2010;21:1440.

# Ongogenic Osteomalacia

- **Essentials of Diagnosis**
  - A paraneoplastic syndrome usually associated with benign mesenchymal tumors.
  - Hypophosphatemia (from increased urinary phosphate excretion), increased alkaline phosphatase, and low levels of 1,25-dihydroxyvitamin D (calcitriol) suggest the diagnosis.
  - Clinical manifestations include fatigue, weakness, bone pain, deformities, and/or recurrent fractures.

- **Differential Diagnosis**
  - Benign mesenchymal tumors (ie, hemangiopericytoma, a phosphoturic mesenchymal tumor, mixed connective tissue type (PMTMCT) is most common—70–80%).
  - Malignant mesenchymal tumors.
  - Other causes of osteomalacia.

- **Treatment**
  - Surgical resection (often curative).
  - Calcitriol and phosphorus supplementation.

- **Pearl**

*Always monitor for hypercalcemia, nephrolithiasis, and nephrocalcinosis when treating long term with high levels of calcitriol and phosphorus supplementation.*

Reference

Jan de Beur SM: Tumor-induced osteomalacia. JAMA. 2005;294:1260.

# Tetany

## ■ Essentials of Diagnosis
- Sensory: perioral and extremity paresthesias.
- Motor: stiffness, cramping, and spasm.
- Autonomic: brochospasm, bile duct spasm, diaphoresis.
- Classic exam findings (not sensitive or specific for hypocalcemia): Trosseau sign (carpopedal spasm during inflation of blood pressure cuff) and Chvostek sign (lipsilateral facial muscle contraction with tapping of cranial nerve VII anterior to the ear).

## ■ Differential Diagnosis
- The most common causes of tetany are hypocalcemia and alkalosis, which result in hyperexcitability of neurons.
- Most commonly occurs when the serum calcium level is less than 7.0–7.5 mg/dL.
- Symptoms also may be exacerbated or caused by hypomagnesemia and hypokalemia.
- Severity of symptoms is related to the rapidity of onset of the underlying metabolic disturbance.

## ■ Treatment
- Intravenous repletion of calcium, magnesium, or potassium deficits.
- Correction of underlying causes of metabolic disturbance, including respiratory or (less commonly) metabolic alkalosis.

## ■ Pearl
*Tetany may be life-threatening so must be treated urgently.*

Reference

Thome et al: Hypocalcemic emergencies. Endocrinol Metabol Clin N Am 1995;79(2):363–375.

# Vitamin D Deficiency

## ■ Essentials of Diagnosis
- Results from inadequate intake, inadequate sunlight exposure, impaired gut absorption, or impaired production and endogenous conversion to active vitamin D metabolites.
- Leads to impaired bone mineralization—rickets in children, osteomalacia in adults, with chronic muscle and bone pain, deformities, and increased fracture risk.
- Diagnosed by measuring calcidiol, or 25-hydroxyvitamin D. Levels less than 15–20 ng/mL are considered deficient.
- Risk factors include the elderly, malnutrition, obesity, darker skin color, and lack of sun exposure.
- PTH, if checked, may be elevated.

## ■ Differential Diagnosis
- Poor nutritional intake.
- Lack of sunlight exposure.
- Malabsorption (celiac disease, short bowel syndrome, cystic fibrosis, pancreatitis, etc).
- End-stage liver disease.
- Medications that accelerate vitamin D metabolism (eg, phenytoin, phenobarbitol).

## ■ Treatment
- Ergocalciferol (vitamin $D_2$) 50,000 IU one to three times per week (depending on severity and etiology) until levels are sufficient (>32 ng/mL)—usually 8–10 weeks.
- Increase sunlight exposure and dietary intake.

## ■ Pearl
*Vitamin D deficiency, when defined as less than 20 ng/mL, is exceedingly common—up to 55–60% of elderly nursing home individuals and hospitalized patients.*

Reference
Holick MF: Vitamin D deficiency. N Engl J Med 2007;357:266.

# Vitamin D Intoxication

- **Essentials of Diagnosis**
  - Hypercalcemia often with hyperphosphatemia.
  - Symptoms include confusion, polyuria, polydipsia, anorexia, vomiting, muscle weakness, bone pain, hearing loss, and/or seizures.
  - May present with renal failure, hypertension, band keratopathy.
  - Laboratory and radiologic findings include hypercalcemia, hypercalciuria, evaluated 25-hydroxyvitamin D levels, hyperphosphatemia, and bone demineralization.

- **Differential Diagnosis**
  - Primary hyperparathyroidism.
  - Hypercalcemia of malignancy.
  - Milk alkali syndrome.
  - Familial hypocalciuric hypercalcemia.
  - Granulomatous disease.
  - Medication-induced hypercalcemia.
  - Immobilization.

- **Treatment**
  - Discontinuation of vitamin D ingestion.
  - Wear sunscreen or avoid exposure to sunlight.
  - Intravenous hydration; and once intravascular resuscitation have occurred, possibly loop diuretics.
  - Glucocorticoids. If severe hypercalcemia, dialysis may be indicated.

- **Pearl**

*Vitamin D intoxication is diagnosed by a thorough clinical history of ingestion of large doses of vitamin D, and may cause multisystem disease.*

References

Jacobus CH et al: Hypervitaminosis D associated with drinking milk. N Engl J Med 1992;326(18):1173.

Koutkia P et al: Vitamin D intoxication associated with an over-the-counter supplement. N Engl J Med 2001;345:66.

# 1.5

# Disorders of Phosphate Metabolism

## Hyperphosphatemia

- **Essentials of Diagnosis**
  - Serum inorganic phosphorous (Pi) concentration greater than 4.5 mg/dL.
  - Occurs due to increased phosphorous intake, decreased renal phosphorous excretion, or transcellular shifts of phosphorous from cells into extracellular fluid space.
  - Acute hyperphosphatemia can cause hypocalcemia and related clinical manifestations including tetany, and sequelae of calcium-phosphate salt deposition in kidneys, heart, blood vessels.
  - Chronic hyperphosphatemia can result in tissue phosphate deposition and secondary hyperparathyroidism (in patients with chronic kidney disease).

- **Differential Diagnosis**
  - Decreased renal excretion: acute or chronic kidney disease, hypoparathyroidism, pseudohypoparathyroidism, tumoral calcinosis.
  - Increased phosphorous intake: usually requires reduced renal excretion, phosphate-containing laxatives and enemas, parenteral nutrition, vitamin D toxicity.
  - Release of phosphorous from cells: tumor lysis syndrome, rhabdomyolysis, severe hemolytic anemia, acute leukemia, fulminant hepatic necrosis.

- **Treatment**
  - Directed at the cause of the hyperphosphatemia.
  - If occurring at reduced GFR, treatment should also include decreased intake and use of oral phosphate binders.
  - If severe, acute, and refractory to other treatments, then dialysis may be required.
  - Calcimimetics (cinacalcet) may be used in secondary hyperparathyroidism of chronic kidney disease.

- **Pearl**

*Severe acute hyperphosphatemia can occur with use of sodium phosphate laxatives and enemas; and can cause severe acute hypocalcemia, acute phosphate nephropathy, and death.*

References

Markowitz GS, Perazella MA: Acute phosphate nephropathy. Kidney Int 2009;76:1027.

Molony DA, Stephens BW: Derangements in phosphate metabolism in chronic kidney diseases/endstage renal disease: therapeutic considerations. Adv Chronic Kidney Dis 2011;18:120.

## Hypophosphatemia

- **Essentials of Diagnosis**
  - Defined as a serum inorganic phosphate (Pi ) concentration <1.0 mg/ dL. Pi concentration 1.0–2.5 mg/dL is usually asymptomatic.
  - Clinical manifestations include muscle weakness or paralysis, bone disease, hemolysis, increased risk of infection depending on severity and chronicity.
  - Frequently encountered among alcoholic patients with other electrolyte abnormalities and patients with nutritionally deficient states such as anorexia nervosa and malabsorption.
  - Can occur acutely in patients with acute respiratory alkalosis due to intracellular shift of phosphate.
  - Also occurs in association with severe illness, diabetic ketoacidosis, sepsis, extensive burns.

- **Differential Diagnosis**
  - Decreased phosphorous intake or intestinal absorption: vitamin D deficiency (with rickets in children and osteomalacia in adults), vitamin D-resistant rickets, use of phosphate-binding antacids or calcium supplements, intestinal disorders with malabsoption of Pi and vitamin D, malnutrition, alcoholism.
  - Increased renal phosphate excretion: primary hyperparathyroidism, Fanconi syndrome (primary or drug/toxin related), alcoholism, treatment of ketoacidosis, x-linked hypophosphatemic rickets, autosomal dominant hypophosphatemic rickets, oncogenic osteomalacia.
  - Transcellular shifts of inorganic phosphate: respiratory alkalosis, extensive burns, leukemia blast crisis, refeeding syndrome, insulin administration.

- **Treatment**
  - Treat underlying cause.
  - Mild hypophosphatemia can be treated with oral replacement (eg, milk, other dairy products, sodium- and potassium phosphate salts).
  - More severe hypophosphatemia should be treated with intravenous sodium or potassium phosphate supplementation.

- **Pearl**

*Acute respiratory alkalosis can cause rapid development of profound hypophosphatemia that will spontaneously correct when the respiratory alkalosis resolves and does not generally require any specific treatment.*

Reference

Amanzadeh J, Reilly RF Jr: Hypophosphatemia: an evidence-based approach to its clinical consequences and management. Nat Clin Prac Nephrol 2006;2:136.

# Hypophosphatemic Rickets

## ■ Essentials of Diagnosis

- Vitamin D-dependent (or resistant) rickets (VDDR) type I is due to mutations in the renal *1-alpha hydroxylase* gene with deficiency of active vitamin D. Type II VDDR is due to defects in the vitamin D receptor with resistance to the effects of vitamin D. Both are autosomal recessive.
- X-linked hypophosphatemic rickets (XLHR) involves mutation in the *PHEX* gene that encodes a peptidase that degrades phosphaturic factors ("phosphatonins") such as FGF-23.
- Autosomal dominant hypophosphatemic rickets (ADHR) is due to gain-of-function mutations in the gene encoding FGF-23 leading to its overexpression.

## ■ Differential Diagnosis

- VDDR I and II have hypocalcemia, elevation of alkaline phosphatase and PTH levels, and normal to mildly decreased levels of 25 (OH) vitamin D. 1,25 $(OH)_2$ vitamin D is very low in VDDR I and normal or increased in VDDR II. Bone disease is severe and motor retardation, delayed growth, myopathy, and dental enamel hypoplasia are usually present in VDDR I.
- XLHR and ADHR have phosphaturia and severe hypophosphatemia with normal calcium and PTH levels. 25 (OH) vitamin D levels are normal and 1,25 $(OH)_2$ vitamin D levels are normal or mildly decreased. XLHR is associated with delayed growth. ADHR is associated with muscle weakness and often less significant bone manifestations.

## ■ Treatment

- VDDR I requires large doses of vitamin D but can also be managed with more physiologic doses of calcitriol. VDDR II is treated with large doses of calcium supplementation.
- XLH and ADHR are treated with oral phosphorous replacement and large doses of calcitriol.

## ■ Pearl

*These disorders can usually be diagnosed on clinical grounds and with testing of calcium, PTH, and 25 (OH) vitamin D levels so that testing for 1,25 $(OH)_2$ vitamin D is usually not necessary.*

References

Alizadeh Naderi AS, Reilly RF: Hereditary disorders of renal phosphate wasting. Nat Rev Nephrol 2010;6:657.

Tenenhouse HS, Murer H: Disorders of renal tubular phosphate transport. J Am Soc Nephrol 2003;14:240.

# 1.6

# Disorders of Magnesium Metabolism

## Hypermagnesemia

- **Essentials of Diagnosis**
  - Serum magnesium concentration greater than 2.5 mg/dL (2.1 mEq/L).
  - Patients are usually asymptomatic until the serum Mg exceeds 4–5 mg/dL; clinical manifestations at higher levels include:
    - 5–7 mg/dL: hyporeflexia, nausea, vomiting, flushing.
    - 7–12 mg/dL: loss of deep tendon reflexes, respiratory depression, lethargy, hypotension, EKG changes (prolonged PR, QRS, and QT intervals), hypocalcemia.
    - More than 12 mg/dL: apnea, paralysis, coma, complete heart block, asystole.

- **Differential Diagnosis**
  - Hypermagnesemia occurs primarily in patients with impaired renal magnesium excretion capacity due to advanced CKD or acute renal failure. These patients are vulnerable to severe and potentially fatal hypermagnesemia when exposed to a high magnesium load, which may be endogenous (eg, tumor lysis, rhabdomyolysis) or exogenous (eg, ingestion of Mg-containing laxatives and antacids).
  - Rarely, hypermagnesemia can develop in patients with normal renal function; examples include treatment of preeclampsia with large doses of $MgSO_4$, massive oral ingestions, and chronic laxative abuse.
  - Some disorders cause increased renal magnesium absorption, including hypothyroidism, adrenal insufficiency, hyperparathyroidism, and familial hypocalciuric hypercalcemia.

- **Treatment**
  - Discontinue any source of exogenous magnesium.
  - If severe cardiovascular, neurologic, or respiratory complications are present, administer IV calcium chloride or calcium gluconate to antagonize the effects of magnesium.
  - In patients with normal renal function who are not volume overloaded, volume expansion may enhance renal magnesium excretion; loop diuretics can further augment magnesuria.
  - Patients with renal failure may require dialysis for Mg removal.

- **Pearl**

*It is important to monitor calcium levels when using loop diuretics to treat hypermagnesemia, since these agents can cause hypercalciuria and hypocalcemia, which in turn exacerbates the clinical effects of hypermagnesemia.*

Reference

Topf JM, Murray PT: Hypomagnesemia and hypermagnesemia. Rev Endocr Metab Disord 2003;4(2):195.

# Hypomagnesemia

- **Essentials of Diagnosis**
  - Serum Mg concentration more than 1.5 mg/dL (1.3 mEq/L).
  - May be asymptomatic, especially if mild and slowly developing.
  - The clinical manifestations of severe hypomagnesemia include:.
    - Cardiovascular: arrhythmias (eg, torsade de pointes, ventricular fibrillation), magnification of digitalis toxicity, EKG changes (PR prolongation, QRS widening, T wave changes).
    - Neuromuscular: muscle weakness, fasciculations and cramps, tremor, Chvostek and Trousseau signs, tetany, coma, seizures.
    - Electrolyte disturbances: hypocalcemia, hypokalemia.

- **Differential Diagnosis**
  - Renal Mg wasting: diagnosed by a 24-hour urinary Mg excretion greater than 10–30 mg or fractional excretion of Mg greater than 2% in the setting of hypomagnesemia. Causes include polyuric states, ECF volume expansion, acquired tubular dysfunction, hereditary Mg-wasting disorders, medications (eg, diuretics, cisplatin), hypercalcemia. See separate topic for more details.
  - GI losses: diarrhea (particularly if associated with fat malabsorption), GI fistulas, small bowel resection, or bypass.
  - Redistribution into the intracellular compartment: refeeding syndrome, insulin therapy, metabolic alkalosis.
  - The etiology of hypomagnesemia is often multifactorial in alcoholics and diabetics, particularly in the setting of DKA.

- **Treatment**
  - If hypomagnesemia is severe (< 1.2 mg/dL or 1.0 mEq/L) or symptomatic, administer a 1–2 g bolus of parenteral magnesium sulfate over 15 minutes, followed by a continuous infusion of 4–6 g $MgSO_4$ per 24 hours. Repletion should continue for 1–2 days after serum Mg normalizes. These doses should be reduced in patients with decreased renal function.
  - Use oral magnesium salts (preferably sustained release formulations) for asymptomatic patients or those who need maintenance therapy due to chronic Mg losses.
  - Potassium-sparing diuretics may be beneficial if renal Mg wasting persists despite high-dose oral replacement.

- **Pearl**

*Normomagnesemic Mg depletion should be suspected in patients at risk for Mg depletion who have clinical features consistent with Mg deficit (eg, hypokalemia, hypocalcemia).*

Reference
Agus ZS: Hypomagnesemia. J Am Soc Nephrol 1999;10(7):1616.

## Renal Magnesium Wasting

### ■ Essentials of Diagnosis

- Hypomagnesemia (serum Mg < 1.5 mg/dL or 1.3 mEq/L).
- Inappropriately high renal Mg excretion, as evidenced by either of the following:
  - ○ 24-hour urine collection showing greater than 10–30 mg of magnesium excreted.
  - ○ Fractional excretion of Mg ($FE_{Mg}$) greater than 2%. $FE_{Mg}$ is calculated as follows: (urine Mg × plasma Mg)/(0.7 × plasma Mg × urine Cr) × 100.

### ■ Differential Diagnosis

- Medications:
  - ○ Loop and thiazide diuretics: frequent cause of renal Mg wasting.
  - ○ Cisplatin: causes Mg wasting in more than 50% of patients.
  - ○ Other drugs include aminoglycosides, cyclosporine, pentamidine, amphotericin B.
- Sustained ECF volume expansion (causing increased urinary sodium excretion, which in turn causes magnesium wasting): primary hyperaldosteronism, administration of large amounts of normal saline.
- Polyuric states: uncontrolled hyperglycemia with glucosuria, post-ATN diuresis, postobstructive diuresis, polyuria after renal transplantation.
- Other electrolyte disturbances: hypercalcemia, hypokalemia, and phosphate depletion inhibit tubular Mg reabsorption.
- Inherited disorders of renal Mg handling (rare):
  - ○ Diseases affecting the thick ascending limb of the loop of Henle (eg, Bartter syndrome): associated with hypercalciuria and hypocalcemia, and sometimes with hypokalemia.
  - ○ Diseases affecting the distal convoluted tubule (eg, Gitelman syndrome): associated with low or normal urinary calcium.

### ■ Treatment

- Correction of the cause of Mg wasting whenever possible.
- Mg repletion using parenteral Mg for severe or symptomatic hypomagnesemia, and oral Mg for maintenance therapy in patients with chronic losses (see section on Hypomagnesemia).
- Potassium-sparing diuretics (eg, spironolactone, amiloride) if hypomagnesemia persists despite high-dose oral replacement.

### ■ Pearl

*The finding of hypermagnesuria and hypocalciuria suggests impaired distal convoluted tubule function.*

Reference

Konrad M, Weber S: Recent advances in molecular genetics of hereditary magnesium-losing disorders. J Am Soc Nephrol 2003;14:249.

# 1.7

# Acid-Base Disorders

## Ethylene Glycol Poisoning

### ■ Essentials of Diagnosis
- Cause of elevated anion gap acidosis.
- Can be rapidly lethal.
- Found in antifreeze.
- Metabolized by alcohol dehydrogenase to glycolic acid, and other toxic byproducts.
- Causes increased osmolar gap.
- Calculated serum osmolarity: $2\,[Na^+] + [glucose]/18 + [BUN]/2.8$.
- Elevated osmol gap: measured – calculated osmolol greater than 10.
- Can cause renal failure with oxalate crystals.

### ■ Differential Diagnosis
- Elevated osmolar gap commonly seen in methanol, ethylene glycol, and alcoholic ketoacidosis.
- Slight osmolar gap may be seen in lactic acidosis and chronic renal failure.
- Ethylene glcyol's metabolism can cause renal failure whereas methanol's metabolism affects vision.

### ■ Treatment
- Infusion of ethanol.
- Infusion of fomepizole (competitive inhibitor of alcohol dehydrogenase).
- Hemodialysis.

### ■ Pearl
*Propylene glycol is a solution through which certain drips in the ICU are delivered, including lorazepam, which can sometimes cause anion gap acidosis with increased serum osmolality.*

Reference

Brent J: Fomepizole for ethylene glycol and methanol poisoning. N Engl J Med 2009;360:2216.

## Isopropyl Alcohol Poisoning

- **Essentials of Diagnosis**
  - Isopropyl alcohol is commonly included in disinfectants, rubbing alcohol, and solvents.
  - Laboratory tests reveal a high osmolar gap, created by both the isopropyl alcohol and its metabolite acetone.
  - Does not cause acidosis or elevated anion gap.
  - Other supportive lab data include elevated serum and urine ketones.
  - Clinical symptoms include altered mental status similar to ethanol intoxiciation, nausea, vomiting, and fruity breath odor.

- **Differential Diagnosis**
  - Methanol and ethylene glycol ingestion.
  - Diabetic ketoacidosis.
  - Alcoholic ketoacidosis.
  - Acetone ingestion.

- **Treatment**
  - Typically requires observation and supportive care alone.
  - Rarely, massive ingestion can cause hemodynamic instability which requires hemodialysis.
  - No role for antidote therapy as the metabolite acetone is less toxic than isopropyl alcohol itself.

- **Pearl**

*Unlike methanol and ethylene glycol ingestion, isopropyl toxicity is from the parent compound and presents with an osmolar gap without metabolic acidosis.*

Reference

Abramson S, Singh AK: Treatment of the alcohol intoxications: ethylene glycol, methanol, and isopropanol. Curr Opin Nephrol Hypertens 2000;9:695.

# Ketoacidosis

## ■ Essentials of Diagnosis
- Common cause of an elevated anion gap acidosis.
- Typically precipitated by diabetes or alcohol abuse.
- Diabetic ketoacidosis (DKA) typically has history of noncompliance or precipitant such as infection or MI.
- DKA is classically seen in type I diabetes.
- Alcoholic ketoacidosis (AKA) classically presents in a patient on alcohol binge that has nausea, vomiting, and decreased oral intake.

## ■ Differential Diagnosis
- DKA: characterized by hyperglycemia, acidemia, positive nitroprusside reaction test.
- In some cases of DKA, nitroprusside may be negative reflecting predominance of β-hydroxybutyrate over acetate.
- AKA: characterized by hypoglycemia, positive nitroprusside reaction test, milder acidemia compared to DKA.
- AKA may also present elevated serum osmolal gap.

## ■ Treatment
- DKA: fluid resuscitation, insulin administration, correction of potassium deficits.
- AKA: volume repletion, administration of glucose after or with thiamine administration, electrolyte repletion.

## ■ Pearl
*Patients with DKA often have total body potassium depletion but elevated serum potassium and need frequent potassium monitoring and replacement during the management of DKA.*

Reference

Casteels K: Diabetic ketoacidosis. Rev Endocr Metab Disord 2003;4:159.

## Lactic Acidosis

- **Essentials of Diagnosis**
  - Common cause of acute metabolic acidosis.
  - Likely most frequent cause of severe metabolic acidosis as defined by blood pH less than 7.1, plasma bicarbonate less than 8–10 mEq/L.
  - Diagnosed by serum lactate greater than 5 mEq/L.
  - Anaerobic metabolism results in the production of lactic acid.

- **Differential Diagnosis**
  - Type A lactic acidosis: associated with tissue hypoxia and readily suspected by presence of hypotension and reduced tissue perfusion.
    - Examples: severe hypoxemia, vigorous exercise, profound anemia, shock, mesenteric ischemia, massive PE, severe heart failure.
  - Type B lactic acidosis: typically normal oxygen delivery and often a result of several medications.
    - Examples include: metformin, nucleoside analogues.
  - D lactic acidosis: needs to be specifically measured by a separate assay, commonly seen in short gut syndrome after high carbohydrate load.

- **Treatment**
  - Treat the underlying cause (eg, sepsis or withdrawal of medication).

- **Pearl**

*There is much controversy surrounding administration of bicarbonate in severe academia as it may paradoxically lower intracellular pH.*

Reference

Gauthier PM, Szerlip HM: Metabolic acidosis in the intensive care unit. Crit Care Clin 2002;18:289

# Metabolic Acidosis with Elevated Anion Gap

## ■ Essentials of Diagnosis

- Metabolic acidosis caused principally by the reduction of plasma bicarbonate concentration.
- Anion gap calculated by: $Na^+ - (Cl^- + HCO_3^-)$. Normal ~10–12 mEq/L.
- Increase in serum anion gap usually the result of retention of unmeasured anions typically due to addition of organic acid.
- The respiratory response to metabolic acidosis is increased alveolar ventilation, manifested by decrease in $Pco_2$.
- For every 10 mEq/L decrease in $HCO_3$, $Pco_2$ should drop by approximately 12 mm Hg.

## ■ Differential Diagnosis

- Renal failure: acute or chronic.
- Diabetic ketoacidosis.
- Alcoholic ketoacidosis.
- Lactic acidosis.
- Salicylate intoxication typically with concominant respiratory alkalosis.
- Methanol poisoning.
- Ethylene glycol poisoning.

## ■ Treatment

- Reversal of the cause.
- Though controversial, bicarbonate infusion if blood pH less than 7.1.
- In treatment of chronic metabolic acidosis, as in chronic renal failure, oral bicarbonate repletion or products metabolized into bicarbonate (ie, sodium citrate).

## ■ Pearl

*The normal serum anion gap will decrease by ~2.5 mEq/L for each 1 g/dL drop in serum albumin.*

### Reference

Reilly RF, Anderson RJ: Interpreting the anion gap. Crit Care Med 1998;26:1771.

## Metabolic Acidosis with Normal Anion Gap

- **Essentials of Diagnosis**
  - Metabolic acidosis is a process that lowers plasma bicarbonate and results in a decrease in blood pH.
  - Appropriate respiratory compensation causes a lowering of $PCO_2$.
  - Anion Gap is calculated by $Na^+ - (Cl^- + HCO_3)$. Normal gap is ~10–12.
  - A metabolic acidosis with a normal anion gap is associated with elevated chloride levels and often referred to as the hyperchloremic metabolic acidosis.

- **Differential Diagnosis**
  - Gastrointestinal causes of bicarbonate loss: diarrhea, intestinal fistula, pancreatic fistula, ileal conduit.
  - Renal causes: proximal renal tubular acidosis (renal loss of bicarbonate), distal renal tubular acidosis (decreased renal excretion of $H^+$).

- **Treatment**
  - Identify and treat the underlying cause.
  - Treatment of acute metabolic acidosis is controversial, but recommended with bicarbonate infusion for pH less than 7.1.
  - Monitor ionized calcium levels during acute bicarbonate supplementation.
  - Treatment of chronic metabolic acidosis with oral bicarbonate supplementation is indicated for maintenance of normal bone and muscle metabolism.

- **Pearl**

*Metabolic acidosis with a normal anion gap often results from gastrointestinal and renal diseases, which lower serum bicarbonate levels.*

Reference

Kraut JA, Madias NE: Serum anion gap: its uses and limitations in clinical medicine. Clin J Am Soc Nephrol 2007;2:162.

## Metabolic Alkalosis

- **Essentials of Diagnosis**
  - Increase in plasma [$HCO_3^-$].
  - Compensatory increase in arterial $PCO_2$.
  - Increase in arterial pH.

- **Differential Diagnosis**
  - Chloride depletion (urinary [K] <20 mEq/L): gastrointestinal losses (vomiting or nasogastric aspiration, congenital chloridorrhea, villous adenoma), renal losses (chloruretic diuretics, posthypercapnia, severe potassium depletion), and skin losses in cystic fibrosis.
  - Potassium losses: gastrointestinal losses (laxative abuse), renal losses (hyperaldosteronism [primary and secondary] other hypokalemic hypertensive syndromes, Bartter and Gitelman syndromes).
  - Miscellaneous (low glomerular filtration rate with base loading, milk-alkali syndrome, hypercalcemia, nonreabsorbable antacids with cation exchange resin, hypoalbuminemia and recovery from starvation).
  - Transient (multiple blood transfusions with citrate, infant formulas with low chloride content).

- **Treatment**
  - Specific treatment needed when pH greater than 7.55 or $HCO_3$ greater than 33 mEq/L.
  - Both volume depletion and hypokalemia must be corrected.
  - Chloride-depletion alkalosis: if volume contracted, first replete volume with normal saline then replete K with KCl. If volume expanded, give KCl alone. Dialysis is effective in ESRD.
  - Treat or reverse causative factors: stop diuretics (or add K-sparing agent, especially in hyperaldosteronism) and alkali therapy, reduce GI loss of acid and K.
  - Potassium depletion: oral KCl.
  - In severe cases, HCl administration through a central venous catheter or ammonium chloride, should be considered.
  - If volume overloaded, acetazolamide 250–500 mg/day orally can be used to promote bicarbonate loss. This is most effective if used with other diuretics but can cause severe hypokalemia.

- **Pearl**

*TTKG of greater than 4 with hypokalemia suggests renal K wasting.*

Reference
Galla JH: Metabolic alkalosis. J Am Soc Nephrol 2000;11:369.

# Metabolic Alkalosis with Normal or Low Blood Pressure

## ■ Essentials of Diagnosis
- Acid-base disorder with primary accumulation of base or net loss of acid.
- Diagnosed with increase in plasma [$HCO_3^-$] and compensatory increase in blood pH in setting of normal to low DP.
- Should be compensatory increase in $CO_2$ (hypoventilation).
- Serum potassium concentration is usually low.

## ■ Differential Diagnosis
- Diuretic therapy.
- Vomiting, NG aspiration.
- Cystic fibrosis.
- Post hypercapnia.
- Bartter syndrome.
- Gitelman syndrome.
- Congenital chloidorrhea.
- Milk-alkali syndrome.

## ■ Treatment
- Correction of the underlying disturbance.
- If ECF volume contracted, replace with isotonic saline.
- Replace potassium deficiency.

## ■ Pearl
*Bartter and Gitelman syndromes can mimic surreptitious loop and thiazide diuretic abuse, respectively.*

Reference
Galla JH: Metabolic alkalosis. J Am Soc Nephrol 2000;11:369.

# Metabolic Alkalosis with Normal Urine Chloride

## ■ Essentials of Diagnosis
- Acid-base disorder with accumulation of base or net loss of acid.
- Diagnosed with increase in plasma [$HCO_3^-$] and increase in blood pH.
- Should be compensatory increase with $P_{CO_2}$ (hypoventilation).
- Urine [$Cl^-$] greater than 20 mEq/L suggests $K^+$ depletion alkalosis or other miscellaneous disorders not primarily due to ECF volume contraction and usually associated with hypokalemia.
- Physical examination is helpful for assessing the extracellular fluid status.

## ■ Differential Diagnosis
- Diuretics use.
- Hyperaldosteronism, hypercortisolism.
- Bartter and Gitelman syndromes.
- Low GFR with base loading.
- Milk-alkali syndrome.
- Hypercalcemia (rare).
- Non-reabsorbable antacid with cation exchange resin.
- Hypoalbuminemia (mild).

## ■ Treatment
- Treat hypokalemia with KCl.
- In case of mineralocorticoid or cortisol excess, blockade or removal of the source. Medical blockade includes $K^+$-sparing diuretics.

## ■ Pearl
*In metabolic alkalosis, determination of the volume status assists in determination of primary diagnosis.*

Reference

Galla JH: Metabolic alkalosis. J Am Soc Nephrol 2000;11:369.

## Metabolic Alkalosis with Low Urine Chloride

- **Essentials of Diagnosis**
  - Acid-base disorder with accumulation of base or net loss of acid in setting of volume ECF volume contraction.
  - Diagnosed with increase in plasma $[HCO_3^-]$ and increase in blood pH.
  - Should be compensatory to increase in $P_{CO_2}$ (hypoventilation).
  - Urine $[Cl^-]$ less than 20 mEq/L as indication of ECF in volume depletion.

- **Differential Diagnosis**
  - GI losses: vomiting, nasogastric aspiration, congenital chloridorrhea, villous adenoma.
  - Renal losses: diuretics (in chronic state), posthypercapnia, severe hypokalemia.
  - Skin losses: cystic fibrosis.

- **Treatment**
  - If ECF volume contracted, replace with normal saline.
  - Replace potassium deficit with potassium chloride (KCl).
  - If alkalosis is severe and not readily reversible, HCl (0.1 N) can be given.

- **Pearl**

*Urine $[Cl^-]$ is used as indication/effective intravascular volume instead of urine $[Na^+]$.*

Reference

Galla JH: Metabolic alkalosis. J Am Soc Nephrol 2000;11:369.

## Metabolic Alkalosis with High Blood Pressure

■ **Essentials of Diagnosis**
- Acid-base disorder with accumulation of base or net loss of acid.
- Increase in plasma [$HCO_3^-$] and increase in blood pH with compensatory increase in $Pco_2$ (hypoventilation).
- Typically associated with urine [$Cl^-$] greater than 20 mEq/L.
- Often associated with hypokalemia.
- Urine $K^+$ excretion greater than 30 mEq/day in the presence of hypokalemia suggests mineralocorticoid excess.

■ **Differential Diagnosis**
- Primary hyperaldosteronism.
- Renal artery stenosis.
- Liddle syndrome.
- Licorice ingestion.
- Cushing syndrome.
- Primary deoxycorticosterone excess: $11\beta$ and $17\alpha$ hydroxylase deficiency.

■ **Treatment**
- $K^+$-sparing diuretics.
- Replace KCl.

■ **Pearl**
*Patients with primary aldosteronism typically have an aldosterone to renin ratio more than 20.*

Reference

Khosla N, Hogan D: Mineralocorticoid hypertension and hypokalemia. Semin Nephrol 2006;26:434.

## Methanol Poisoning

- **Essentials of Diagnosis**
  - Elevated anion gap acidosis due to metabolism and formic acid.
  - Increased osmolar gap, which declines as methanol is metabolized.
  - Optic papillitis.

- **Differential Diagnosis**
  - Elevated osmolar gap commonly seen in methanol, ethylene glycol, and alcoholic ketoacidosis.
  - Slight osmolar gap may be seen in lactic acidosis and chronic renal failure.
  - Methanol's metabolites affect the eyes, whereas ethylene glycol's affect the kidneys (calcium oxalate crystals).

- **Treatment**
  - Infusion of fomepizole (competitive inhibitor of alcohol dehydrogenase).
  - Infusion of ethanol.
  - Hemodialysis.

- **Pearl**

*If ethanol is also present, its contribution to the osmolar gap is estimated by dividing its concentration in mg/dL by 4.6.*

Reference

Brent J: Fomepizole for ethylene glycol and methanol poisoning. N Engl J Med 2009;360:2216.

# Renal Tubular Acidosis, Distal with Hyperkalemia

## ■ Essentials of Diagnosis
- Caused by decreased secretion of $H^+$ from the distal nephron.
- Due to either aldosterone deficiency or tubular resistance to aldosterone, which leads to hyperkalemia.
- Typically results in milder acidosis as compared to distal RTA with hypokalemia.
- Causes of aldosterone deficiency include: adrenal insufficiency, congenital adrenal hyperplasia, diabetic nephropathy, ACE-inhibitors, NSAIDs, calcineurin inhibitors, multiple myeloma.
- Causes of aldosterone resistance: amiloride, spironolactone, triamterene, trimethaprim, pentamidine, tubulointerstitial disease, pseudohypoaldosteronism, urinary tract obstruction.

## ■ Differential Diagnosis
- Renal insufficiency.

## ■ Treatment
- Fludrocortisone can be used to treat aldosterone deficiency but side effects include elevated blood pressure and fluid overload.
- Low potassium diet and diuretics.

## ■ Pearl
*Most common cause is acquired hyporeninemic hypoaldosteronism seen in diabetics.*

Reference

Rodriguez Soriano J: Renal tubular acidosis: the clinical entity. J Am Soc Nephrol 2002;13:2160.

# Renal Tubular Acidosis, Distal with Normal or Low Potassium

- **Essentials of Diagnosis**
  - Caused by decreased $H^+$ secretion by the distal nephron.
  - Can have very low serum bicarbonate levels (<10 mEq/L).
  - Urine pH greater than 5.5.
  - Major causes include: primary (idiopathic), familial autosomal dominant or recessive, Sjögren syndrome, hypercalciuria, rheumatoid arthritis, hyperglobulinemia, amphotericin B, cirrhosis, systemic lupus erythematosus, lithium carbonate, sickle cell anemia.
  - Common complication is kidney stones due to increased urinary calcium excretion.

- **Differential Diagnosis**
  - Proximal renal tubular acidosis.
  - Gastrointestinal bicarbonate losses.

- **Treatment**
  - Bicarbonate replacement, usually potassium citrate, to correct both the acidosis and hypokalemia.
  - Less bicarbonate supplementation is required compared to patients with proximal renal tubular acidosis disorders.

- **Pearl**

*Type I RTA can rarely be the presenting symptom of an autoimmune disease such as Sjögren syndrome and rheumatoid arthritis.*

Reference

Rodriguez Soriano J: Renal tubular acidosis: the clinical entity. J Am Soc Nephrol 2002;13:2160.

# Renal Tubular Acidosis, Proximal

## ■ Essentials of Diagnosis
- Caused by impaired proximal tubule reabsorption of filtered $HCO_3^-$ leading to urinary bicarbonate wasting.
- Hyperchloremic normal anion gap metabolic acidosis.
- Urine pH greater than 5.5 in acute phase or when patient is given bicarbonate supplementation.
- Urine pH less than 5.5 in the chronic steady state.
- Fractional excretion of $HCO_3$ is elevated (>20%) in acute phase or when patient is given bicarbonate supplementation.
- Usually associated with low or normal serum potassium.
- Common causes include: multiple myeloma, ifosfamide, amyloidosis, heavy metals, inherited disorders such as cystinosis, tyrosinemia, galactosemia, and Wilson disease.

## ■ Differential Diagnosis
- Carbonic anhydrase inhibitor use.
- Distal renal tubular acidosis.
- Diarrhea.
- Ileal Diversion.

## ■ Treatment
- Sodium bicarbonate (such as sodium or potassium citrate) supplementation to maintain serum bicarbonate greater than 20 mmol/L.
- In children, should maintain serum bicarbonate greater than 22 mmol/L.
- Typically requires high dose of bicarbonate to replace urinary losses of bicarbonate (>5–10 mmol/kg/day).
- Supplement potassium as needed.

## ■ Pearl
*Acquired proximal RTA in adults, especially associated with other proximal tubule reabsorptive defects such as glucosuria, phosphaturia, uricosuria, and aminoaciduria (Fanconi syndrome) must consider multiple myeloma.*

Reference

Rodriguez Soriano J: Renal tubular acidosis: the clinical entity. J Am Soc Nephrol 2002;13:2160.

## Respiratory Acidosis

- **Essentials of Diagnosis**
  - A result of hypoventilation from any cause.
  - On an arterial blood gas, high $P_{CO_2}$, and low pH.
  - Acute respiratory acidosis: $HCO_3$ rises by 1 mEq/L for each 10 mm Hg rise in $P_{CO_2}$.
  - Chronic respiratory acidosis: $HCO_3$ rises by 4 mEq/L for each 10 mm Hg rise in $P_{CO_2}$.
  - If observed $HCO_3$ compensation is too little or too much compared to the predicted $HCO_3$ level, another acid-base abnormality (a mixed disorder) must be present.

- **Differential Diagnosis**
  - Airway: laryngospasm, foreign body aspiration, obstructive sleep apnea.
  - Pulmonary: asthma, severe pulmonary edema, severe pneumonia, COPD, interstitial lung disease, obstructive sleep apnea, ARDS with poor lung compliance, excess oxygen administration in patients with chronic hypercapnia.
  - Drugs: anxiolytics, opiates, neuromuscular blockers.
  - Neurologic: Guillain-Barre, myasthenia gravis, poliomyelitis, diaphragmatic paralysis, amyotrophic lateral sclerosis.
  - Other: flail chest, kyphoscoliosis, obesity, hypoventilation syndrome.

- **Treatment**
  - Identify and treat underlying cause.
  - May require mechanical ventilation in acute respiratory acidosis to treat dangerous levels of acidemia.
  - Rarely patients with chronic respiratory acidosis can be treated with a low carbohydrate diet to decrease $CO_2$ production.

- **Pearl**

*Consider severe hypokalemia and hypophosphatemia as causes of respiratory muscle weakness.*

Reference

Rose BD, Post TW: Clinical physiology of acid-base and electrolyte disorders, 5th ed, McGraw-Hill, New York, 2001, pp. 647.

## Respiratory Alkalosis

■ **Essentials of Diagnosis**
- A result of hyperventilation from any cause.
- On an arterial blood gas, low $P_{CO_2}$ and high pH.
- Acute respiratory alkalosis: $HCO_3$ falls by 2 mEq/L for each 10 mm Hg fall in $P_{CO_2}$.
- Chronic respiratory alkalosis: $HCO_3$ falls by 5 mEq/L for each 10 mm Hg in $P_{CO_2}$.
- If observed $HCO_3$ compensation is too little or too much compared to the predicted $HCO_3$ level, another acid-base abnormality (a mixed disorder) must be present.

■ **Differential Diagnosis**
- Supratentorial: anxiety, pain, fever.
- Pulmonary: pulmonary embolism, hypoxemia, mechanical ventilation, high altitude, pulmonary edema.
- Central nervous system: meningitis, encephalitis, tumor, stroke.
- Drugs: salicylates, progesterone, theophylline, catecholamines, thyroxine.
- Other: pregnancy, sepsis, liver disease, exercise, thyrotoxicosis, alcohol withdrawal.

■ **Treatment**
- Identify and treat underlying cause.
- Often can use anxiolytics, analgesics, and antipyretics.
- Severe alkalosis can cause neuromuscular irritability, including seizures, paresthesias, confusion, and ventricular arrhythmias.

■ **Pearl**

*Unexplained respiratory alkalosis may be a sign of early sepsis.*

**Reference**

Laffey JG, Kavanagh BP: Hypocapnia. N Eng J Med 2002; 347:43.

## Salicylate Toxicity

- **Essentials of Diagnosis**
  - Directly stimulates the respiratory center of the medulla causing a simultaneous respiratory alkalosis.
  - Common clinical complaints include tinnitus, nausea, vomiting, and confusion.
  - Can rarely cause an elevated prothrombin time.

- **Differential Diagnosis**
  - Other ingestions causing high anion gap metabolic acidosis: alcohol, methanol, ethylene glycol.
  - Diabetic ketoacidosis.
  - Lactic acidosis.

- **Treatment**
  - Activated charcoal.
  - Supplemental glucose even if normal serum glucose.
  - Alkalinize both serum and urine. Urine pH goal should be 7.5 to 8.0 to increase excretion.
  - Hemodialysis if altered mental status, pulmonary edema, or renal failure.

- **Pearl**

*Avoid intubation if at all possible as the respiratory alkalosis prevents salicylate anions from crossing the blood brain barrier and causing toxicity.*

**Reference**

Dargan PI et al: An evidence based flowchart to guide the management of acute salicylate (aspirin) overdose. Emerg Med J 2002;19:206.

# 2

# Acute Kidney Injury

## Acute Kidney Injury (AKI)

### ■ Essentials of Diagnosis

- An acute reduction in the glomerular filtration rate (GFR).
- May be also associated with oliguria (urine output <400 mL in 24 hours) or with normal urine output.
- RIFLE (risk, injury, failure, loss, end-stage) criteria consists of various graded levels of kidney injury stratified by urine output and percent rise in kidney function.
- Symptoms: decrease in urine output, dark or cola-colored urine. When severe, anorexia, nausea, malaise, metallic taste, itching, confusion, fluid retention, and hypertension.
- Laboratory studies: serum chemistries, CBC, urinalysis with urine microscopy and urine chemistries. A renal ultrasound to exclude obstruction.
- Urinary findings are often diagnostic of specific etiolgies (muddy brown cast indicative of ATN).
- The fractional excretion of sodium and urea can be utilized in patients with oliguria to determine a prerenal etiology of AKI (FE Na <1% and FE urea <30%).

### ■ Differential Diagnosis

- Prerenal azotemia: most common cause (30–50%) is diminished renal blood flow due to decreased effective arterial blood flow.
- Intrarenal AKI includes: acute tubular necrosis from either nephrotoxins (drugs contrast media, pigments) or ischemia (sepsis); glomerular diseases (glomerulonephritis); interstitial nephritis; and vascular disease.
- Postrenal (obstructive) AKI such as prostatic disease, cervical cancer, retroperitoneal fibrosis.

### ■ Treatment

- Limited, so prevention is critical. Recognition of high-risk patient, avoidance of nephrotoxins, and maintenance of intravascular volume is important.
- Monitor for complications: hyperkalemia, metabolic acidosis, volume overload, hyponatremia, anemia, hyperphosphatemia.
- Prerenal azotemia: reversal of decreased effective renal blood flow (fluids, inotropes).
- Postrenal azotemia: reversal of urinary tract obstruction.
- Dialysis may be required for severe AKI.

### ■ Pearl

*AKI is a common occurrence in critically-ill patients and is associated with significant morbidity and mortality.*

Reference

Schrier RW et al: Acute renal failure: definitions, diagnosis, pathogenesis, and therapy. J Clin Invest 2004;114:5.

# Acute Kidney Injury due to Angiotensin Converting Enzyme Inhibitor or Angiotensin Receptor Blocker

- **Essentials of Diagnosis**
  - Several conditions depend on efferent arteriolar vasoconstriction to maintain adequate glomerular filtration: volume depletion, vasoconstriction caused by certain drugs (NSAIDS), CKD, illnesses with decreased circulatory volumes (CHF), bilateral renal artery stenosis.
  - ACEI and ARBs selectively dilate the efferent arteriole potentially causing AKI in the conditions listed above.
  - After start of ACEI or ARB, serum creatinine can rise within 2 weeks.
  - ARF is usually reversible provided tubular damage (ATN) has not occurred.
  - Hyperkalemia is often present.

- **Differential Diagnosis**
  - Other causes of prerenal failure (volume depletion, CHF, vasoconstrictive drugs [NSAIDS, cyclosporine]).
  - ATN caused by concomitant use of other nephrotoxic drugs or ischemia.

- **Treatment**
  - If serum creatinine rises more than 30%, a reduction in the dose of the ACEI or ARB can be attempted. If renal function is not improving, the ACEI or ARB should be discontinued.
  - A rise of 20% is accepted as the kidneys should benefit from reversing glomerular hyperfiltration.
  - Treatment of hyperkalemia.
  - Rule out other causes for AKI.

- **Pearl**

*Discontinuation of diuretics prior to initiating ACE inhibitor therapy might prevent significant decline in renal function.*

Reference

Bridoux F et al: Acute renal failure after the use of angiotensin-converting-enzyme inhibitors in patients without renal artery stenosis. Nephrol Dial Transplant 1992;7(2):100.

# Acute Kidney Injury due to Chemotherapy: Carboplatin and Cisplatin

## ■ Essentials of Diagnosis
- Platins accumulate in renal tubular cells and bind proteins that are involved in renal tubular energy production and DNA synthesis.
- Platins can cause polyuria, reduced GFR (30–50%), electrolyte disturbances.
- Distal renal tubular acidosis occurs causing metabolic acidosis, hypokalemia, hypomagnesemia.
- ATN and AIN have also been associated with use of platinum-based drugs.

## ■ Differential Diagnosis
- Prerenal failure.
- ATN (ischemic and toxic).
- AIN (drugs).
- Postrenal (obstruction caused by cancer).

## ■ Treatment/Prevention
- Supportive.
- Discontinuation of platins if possible.
- Avoid concomitant use of other potential nephrotoxic drugs (AG, NSAIDS, iodinated contrast media).
- Prehydration.
- Avoidance of large bolus doses.

## ■ Pearl
*Nephrotoxicity is the primary dose-limiting toxicity of cisplatin and carboplatin.*

### Reference
Meyer KB et al: Cisplatin nephrotoxicity. Miner Electolyte Metab 1994;20(4): 201–213.

## Acute Kidney Injury due to Intravenous Immunoglobulins (IVIG)

- **Essentials of Diagnosis**
  - IVIG products contain sucrose which is reabsorbed in the proximal tubule.
  - Human kidneys lack enzyme to hydrolyze sucrose, osmolality rises and cells swell causing vacuolation and tubular obstruction.
  - This extensive vacuolation of the proximal tubules is consistent with osmotic nephrosis.
  - Renal dysfunction occurs within 7 days of IVIG administration.
  - 40% of patients require dialysis.
  - 15% mortality rate despite dialysis.
  - Mean time to recover: 10 days.

- **Differential Diagnosis**
  - Osmotic nephrosis caused by administration of hydroxyethyl-starch and other sucrose-containing solutions.
  - Severe hemolysis due to IVIG can cause hemoglobinuria and renal failure.
  - Depending on underlying medical problem, other etiologies of AKI need to be ruled out: prerenal failure, ATN (toxic or ischemia), postrenal failure due to obstruction.

- **Treatment**
  - Supportive.
  - Sucrose-containing products, if given, should be infused at a low rate (3 mg sucrose/kg/min), hydration prior to administration.

- **Pearl**

*Increased blood viscosity and deposition of immune complexes may contribute to AKI.*

Reference

Dickenmann M et al: Osmotic nephrosis: acute kidney injury with accumulation of proximal tubular lysosomes due to administaration of exogenous solutes. Am J Kidney Dis 2008;51(3):491.

# Acute Kidney Injury due to Rhabdomyolysis & Myoglobinuria

## ■ Essentials of Diagnosis
- Myoglobinuria as a consequence of rhabdomyolysis is a frequent cause of AKI.
- Large amount of myoglobin released from necrotic muscles in the setting of volume depletion causes ATN.
- Trauma, severe hypokalemia and hypophosphatemia, cocaine use, use of HMG Co-A reductase inhibitors (statins), prolonged immobility during periods of loss of consciousness can cause rhabdomyolysis.
- Dark-brown-color urine and muscle pain are common.

## ■ Differential Diagnosis
- Prerenal AKI (bland urine sediment and low $FE_{Na}$).
- Ischemic ATN (evidence of low ECV).
- Obtructive nephropathy (hydronephrosis on ultrasound).
- Diagnosis: positive blood on the urine dipstick, no RBCs.
- Very high serum creatine phosphokinase.
- $FE_{Na}$ greater than 2% and $FE_{Urea}$ greater than 35%, dense granular (muddy brown) casts.
- Hyperkalemia, hyperphosphatemia, hyperuricemia, and hypocalcemia are possible.

## ■ Treatment
- Rapid volume expansion and maintaining high urine flow.
- Early alkalinization of urine.
- Hemodialysis in severe cases.

## ■ Pearl
*Prevention of direct myoglobin-induced tubular toxicity in rhabdomyolysis is possible by early hydration and alkalinization of urine.*

Reference

Bosch X et al: Rhabdomyolysis and acute kidney injury. N Engl J Med 2009;361:62.

## Acute Phosphate Nephropathy

- **Essentials of Diagnosis**
  - Follows use of bowel purgatives that contain oral sodium phosphate (OSP).
  - Acute kidney failure happens days to months after administration of OSP, can lead to CKD.
  - Transient severe hyperphosphatemia (>8 mg/dL) in context of volume depletion leads to precipitation of calcium-phosphorus complexes in tissue, tubular obstruction, and direct tubular epithelial injury.
  - Renal biopsy shows nephrocalcinosis and interstitial nephritis.
  - Risk factors: older age, impaired renal function (CKD), impaired GI-motility, concomitant use of ACEI/ARB/diuretics/NSAIDs.

- **Differential Diagnosis**
  - Acute and chronic tubulointerstitial nephritis of other etiologies.
  - ATN (ischemia or toxins).
  - Tumor lysis syndrome is associated with severe hyperphosphatemia and acute nephrocalcinosis and/or obstruction by uric acid crystals.

- **Treatment**
  - If diagnosed early during phase of AKI and hyperphosphatemia, hemodilaysis can be beneficial.
  - If diagnosed late, patients are treated like patients with CKD.

- **Pearl**

*Acute phosphate nephropathy can occur in normal renal function.*

Reference

Markowitz GS et al: Acute phosphate nephropathy. Kidney Int 2009;76(10):1027.

# Acute Tubular Necrosis, Ischemic

- ■ Essentials of Diagnosis
  - Acute tubular cell injury is the most common cause of intrinsic acute kidney injury (AKI) in the hospital.
  - Progression from prerenal AKI to ischemic acute tubular necrosis (ATN) occurs in four phases: initiation, extension, maintenance, and recovery.
  - Reduced renal blood flow can occur during sepsis, shock, or cardiac surgery.
  - During initiation phase there is injury to the tubular epithelial cells, endothelial cells, and vascular smooth muscle cells due to ATP depletion.
  - In extension phase microvascular congestion, hypoxia, and inflammation are the main events.
  - GFR is at its lowest during maintenance phase. Cells undergo repair during this phase.
  - In the absence of further injury, recovery occurs in 1 to 2 weeks.
  - Acute tubular necrosis (ATN) is usually reversible unless the ischemia was severe enough to cause tubular necrosis.

- ■ Differential Diagnosis
  - Prerenal AKI (bland urine sediment and low $FE_{Na}$).
  - ATN induced by nephrotoxins (history, no evidence of reduced renal perfusion).
  - Acute interstitial nephritis (drugs or infections, high urine eosinophil count, peripheral eosinophilia in some cases and, less commonly, rash and fever).
  - Obstructive nephropathy (ultrasound imaging showing hydronephrosis).
  - $FE_{Na}$ greater than 2% and $FE_{Urea}$ greater than 35%, dense granular (muddy brown) casts, no significant proteinuria or hematuria are helpful in making a diagnosis of ischemic ATN.

- ■ Treatment
  - No specific treatment. In severe cases; hemodialysis.
  - Prevention by treating underlying cause, stabilizing effective circulating volume (ECV), avoiding NSAIDs, ACE inhibitors, and ARB.

- ■ Pearl

*Most common cause of AKI in hospitalized patients, usually reversible, history of low ECV, high $FE_{Na}$, and muddy brown casts in the urine.*

Reference

Rosen S: Acute tubular necrosis is a syndrome of physiologic and pathologic dissociation. J Am Soc Nephrol 2008;19:871.

## Acute Tubular Necrosis (ATN), Nephrotoxic

- **Essentials of Diagnosis**
  - Nephrotoxic agents can cause ATN directly or indirectly.
  - These toxins could be either endogenous or exogenous.
  - Examples of endogenous toxins are hemoglobin and myoglobin.
  - Aminoglycosides (AG), cisplatin, intravenous contrast agents, amphotericin B, pentamidine damage renal tubules directly.
  - Nonsteroidal anti-inflammatory drugs (NSAID, cyclosporine, and intravenous contrast agents) result in tubular ischemia by inducing vasoconstriction.
  - Elderly individuals with diabetes, and those with reduced effective circulating volume (ECV) are at higher risk.
  - AG-induced ATN occurs in 10–20% of patients receiving these drugs for prolonged periods and is usually nonoliguric.
  - Polyuria and hypomagenesemia can be seen in AG-induced ATN.

- **Differential Diagnosis**
  - Prerenal AKI (bland urine sediment and low $FE_{Na}$).
  - Ischemic ATN (evidence of low ECV).
  - Acute interstitial nephritis (drugs or infections, eosinophiluria, and eosinophilia in some cases and, less commonly, rash and fever).
  - Obtructive nephropathy (hydronephrosis on ultrasound).
  - $FE_{Na}$ greater than 2% and $FE_{Urea}$ greater than 35%, dense granular (muddy brown) casts.
  - High serum creatine kinase, positive urine myoglobin suggests ATN due to myoglobinuria.
  - Intravascular hemolysis results in hemoglobinuria, which results in tubular obstruction (low $FE_{Na}$).
  - Positive blood on the dipstick in absence of urine RBCs suggests myoglobinuria or hemoglobinuria.

- **Treatment**
  - No specific treatment, hemodialysis for severe cases.
  - Prevention by avoiding coadministration of multiple toxins, avoiding usage in presence of hypotension, in some cases volume expansion, monitoring serum levels of drugs, limiting the duration of use, avoiding nephrotoxins in patients with reduced GFR.

- **Pearl**

*Old age, reduced GFR, diabetes, and reduced effective circulating volume are risk factors for nephrotoxic ATN.*

Reference

Esson ML, Schrier RW: Diagnosis and treatment of acute tubular necrosis. Ann Intern Med 2002;137:744.

# Aminoglycoside (AG) Nephrotoxicity

## ■ Essentials of Diagnosis
- AG accumulates in renal cortex causing acute tubular necrosis.
- Up to 30% can develop drug-induced concentration defects.
- Often nonoliguric AKI, varies from asymptomatic to irreversible damage requiring lifelong hemodialysis.
- Usual onset is 7–10 days after start of AG.
- Incidence of AG-induced nephrotoxicity is 5–15%.
- Risk factors include old age, preexisting renal impairment, intravascular volume depletion, hepatorenal syndrome, sepsis.
- Renal function returns back to normal level within 2 weeks after discontinuation of the drug, in some cases recovery takes months.

## ■ Differential Diagnosis
- Acute tubular necrosis caused by other nephrotoxic drugs or ischemia.
- Prerenal failure caused by drugs (NSAIDS, diuretics) or states of decreased effective intravascular volumes (sepsis/shock).
- Acute interstitial nephritis (drug induced).
- Tubular obstruction by other drugs.

## ■ Treatment
- Supportive.
- Discontinuation of drug.
- Adjustment of other potential nephrotoxic drugs to reduce renal function.
- Prevention including drug monitoring and short-term treatments is crucial to reduce AG nephrotoxicity.

## ■ Pearl
*Once-daily AG dose maybe less nephrotoxic for a given total daily dose.*

Reference

Pannu N et al: An overview of drug-induced acute kidney injury. Cri Care Med 2008;36(4 Suppl):S216.

## Contrast-Induced Nephropathy (CIN)

- **Essentials of Diagnosis**
  - Rise of serum creatinine greater than 0.5 mg/dL or 25% above baseline creatinine within 48 hours after IV contrast administration.
  - Majority of cases are nonoliguric.
  - Peak in serum creatinine occurs within 3–5 days with complete resolution in 7–10 days for most patients.
  - Oliguria and need for dialysis are unusual and are primarily seen in patients with diabetes with severe chronic kidney disease.
  - CIN is an independent predictor of mortality.
  - Nearly 60% of patients with CIN have significant CKD.

- **Differential Diagnosis**
  - Renal atheroembolism seen in patients receiving contrast arterially (may be accompanied by livedo reticularis, digital ischemia, retinal embolization).
  - Acute tubular necrosis: especially in unstable patients getting contrast studies.
  - Allergic interstitial nephritis: review other medications.
  - Obstructive nephropathy.
  - No specific diagnostic test: urine typically shows signs of tubular necrosis with muddy brown casts. $FE_{Na}$ may initially be less than 1%.

- **Treatment**
  - No specific therapy for CIN.
  - In severe cases may need hemodialysis.
  - Preventative strategies are important and include: mimimize contrast exposure/volume, IV hydration, avoid nephrotoxins (NSAIDS), possibly N-acetylcysteine, and sodium bicarbonate.

- **Pearl**

*CIN occurs predominantly in patients with CKD and preventative strategies are critical as no specific therapy exists.*

Reference

Rudnick MR, Feldman H: Contrast-induced nephropathy: what are the true clinical consequences? Clin J Am Soc Nephrol 2008;3:263.

# Hemolytic Uremic Syndrome (HUS) Associated with Chemotherapeutic Agents

## ■ Essentials of Diagnosis

- HUS is characterized by triad of microangiopathic hemolytic anemia, acute renal failure (thrombotic microangiopathy), and thrombocytopenia.
- HUS is associated with different chemotherapeutic agents: gemcitabine (incidence 0.015%), mitocycin C (incidence 2–10%), cisplatin, bleomycin.
- Chemotherapy can also cause milder forms of hematuria/proteinuria and reduced GFR.
- Mean time between initiation of gentamicin and onset of HUS is about 8 months, other drugs show an association between onset and cumulative dose of drug used.
- Case fatality is high, up to 50–70%.

## ■ Differential Diagnosis

- HUS due to disseminated malignancies.
- HUS after allogeneic hematopoetic cell transplantation.
- HUS due to other drugs: cyclosporine, tacrolimus, quinine, ticlopidine, oral contraceptives.
- HUS due to enterohemorrhagic E. coli, ADAMTS13 deficiency.
- AKI due to ATN (toxic/ischemic), AIN (drugs), or prerenal failure.

## ■ Treatment

- Drug discontinuation.
- Steroids, fresh frozen plasma, hemodilaysis, plasmapheresis, alone or in combination.

## ■ Pearl

*Diagnosis may be delayed as thrombocytopenia and anemia are often attributed to myelotoxicity of chemotherapeutic drug. Increased LDH and schistocytes seen on peripheral blood smear are helpful hints to diagnose HUS/TTP.*

References

Jackson AM et al: Thrombotic microangiopathy and renal failure associated with antineoplastic chemotherapy. Ann Intern Med 1984;101(1):41–44.

Walter RB et al: Gemcitabine-associated hemolytic-uremic syndrome. Am J Kidney Dis 2002;40(4):E16.

# Hepatorenal Syndrome (HRS)

- **Essentials of Diagnosis**
  - Renal failure in patients with advanced liver failure (acute or chronic) in absence of any other causes of renal pathology.
  - Requires exclusion of other causes of renal failure.
  - Characterized by oliguria, severe renal sodium retention, progressive azotemia.
  - Characterized by circulatory instability with systemic arterial vasodilation and activation of vasoactive systems.
  - Type 1: rapid decline in renal function within 2 weeks.
  - Type 2: renal function deteriorates over months.
  - About 50% of patients have some precipitating factors: infection, hemorrhage, overaggressive diuresis, large volume paracentesis.
  - Patients often have stigmata of chronic advanced liver disease.
  - Patients may appear hypovolemic or hypervolemic; and invasive cardiac monitoring to assess intravascular volume may be needed.
  - Serum creatinine may only mildly increase despite severe renal failure due to muscle wasting in cirrhotic patients.

- **Differential Diagnosis**
  - Prerenal azotemia due to volume depletion (diuretics, GI bleeding, large volume paracentesis).
  - Acute tubular necrosis due to ischemia, nephrotoxins.
  - Glomerular diseases associated with liver disease (IgA nephropathy, viral (hepatitis B and C) glomerulonephritis.
  - Differentiation of prerenal azotemia from HRS can be difficult: IV volume challenge to exclude volume depletion.

- **Treatment**
  - All precipitants of hepatorenal syndrome should be reversed.
  - Pharmacotherapy aims to improve systemic hemodynamics.
  - Effective pharmacotherapies include: vasopressin analogues, midodrine, octreotide.
  - Transjugular intrahepatic portosystemic stent shunt (TIPS) has been associated with increase in GFR and renal blood flow.
  - Liver transplantation: GFR may improve even up to 3 months post-transplantation.

- **Pearl**

*Differentiation of hepatorenal syndrome from other etiologies of AKI is critical as the prognosis of hepatorenal syndrome is very poor without liver transplantation.*

Reference

Salerno F et al: Diagnosis, prevention, and treatment of hepatorenal syndrome in cirrhosis. Gut 2007;56:1310.

# Obstructive Uropathy

## ■ Essentials of Diagnosis

- An anatomical or functional problem causes obstruction to the flow of urine in the urinary tract.
- Potential causes include neurogenic bladder, benign prostatic hypertrophy, nephrolithiasis, prostate cancer, cervical cancer, bladder tumors, retroperitoneal fibrosis, retroperitoneal lymphoma, metastatic tumors, and blood clots within the urinary tract.
- Patients can be asymptomatic or present with acute kidney injury (AKI).
- Postrenal AKI should be suspected in the differential diagnosis of acute oliguria and anuria, but many patients do not have reduced urine output.
- 5–10% of AKI cases are post-renal and due to obstruction.

## ■ Differential Diagnosis

- Prerenal AKI (bland urine sediment and low $FE_{Na}$).
- ATN induced by nephrotoxins (history, muddy brown casts).
- Ischemic ATN (evidence of low ECV, muddy brown casts).
- Acute interstitial nephritis (drugs or infections, high urine eosinophil count, peripheral eosinophilia in some cases and less commonly rash and fever).
- Glomrulonephritis (dsymorphic RBCs, RBC casts, heavy proteinuria).
- Renal ultrasound (US) is the diagnostic test of choice (hydronephrosis and possibly hydrouereter).
- High postvoid residual urine volume in the bladder suggests neurogenic bladder or bladder outlet obstruction.
- Negative renal US does not rule out obstructive uropathy.
- Hyperkelemia may be seen in spite of relatively preserved GFR.

## ■ Treatment

- Resolving obstruction by catheterization of the urinary bladder, stent in the ureters, or percutaneous nephrostomy tubes, depending on the level of obstruction, improves GFR in most acute cases.
- In chronic cases, kidneys undergo atrophy and if bilateral and severe, renal replacement therapy may be indicated.

## ■ Pearl

*Renal ultrasound is the diagnostic study of choice.*

Reference

Tseng TY, Stoller ML: Obstructive uropathy. Clin Geriatr Med 2009;25:437.

## Prerenal Azotemia

- **Essentials of Diagnosis**
  - Most common cause of AKI (30–50%).
  - Characterized by decreased effective arterial blood flow either form an absolute reduction in volume of extracellular fluid or in conditions in which effective circulating volume is reduced (heart failure).
  - Physical examination may reveal signs of volume depletion (orthostatic hypotension, dry mucous membranes, flat neck veins) or may demonstrate signs of effective circulating volume depletion (heart failure, edema [third-spacing], cirrhosis).
  - May require invasive testing with measurement of central venous pressure, pulmonary capillary wedge pressure, and cardiac output.
  - Urinary indices-fractional excretion (FE) of sodium and urea can be helpful ($FE_{Na}$ <1%, $FE_{urea}$ <30%).
  - Urine osmolality may be greater than 600 mOsm/kg.
  - May have high serum urea nitrogen/creatinine ratio (>20:1).

- **Differential Diagnosis**
  - Intra-renal causes of AKI (such as acute tubular necrosis, glomerulonephritis, interstitial nephritis, or vascular etiologies).
  - Postrenal (obstructive causes).
  - Note that $FE_{Na}$ less than 1% may be seen in early stages of acute glomerulonephritis, urinary obstruction, pigment nephropathy, and contrast nephropathy.

- **Treatment**
  - In states of true intravascular volume depletion: IV colloid, crystalloid, or blood products as indicated.
  - In states of reduced effective arterial blood flow: attempt to increase renal blood flow through vasoactive drugs (eg, norepinephrine), or inotropic agents (eg, dobutamine).
  - Avoid nonsteroidal anti-inflammatory drugs, ACE-inhibitors, ARBs.
  - Avoid any nephrotoxins.

- **Pearl**

*Prerenal azotemia is the most common form of AKI and if recognized early can be reversed if effective arterial blood flow to the kidney is increased.*

Reference

Kellum JA: Acute kidney injury. Crit Care Med 2008;36(4 suppl):S141.

## Tumor Lysis Syndrome

### ■ Essentials of Diagnosis

- Caused by the rapid release of intracellular contents of tumor cells into the systemic circulation.
- Most commonly seen following treatment of hematologic malignancies with high cellular burden (lymphomas, leukemias).
- Presents with hyperuricemia, hyperkalemia, hyperphosphatemia, hypocalcemia, often accompanied by azotemia, and acute renal failure.
- Dialysis may be required in up to 30% of cases.
- Etiology of renal failure due to acute obstruction of urine flow by precipitated uric acid crystals, as well as acute nephrocalcinosis with interstitial and tubular damage from calcium-phosphorus depostion.
- Presentation depends upon extent of metabolic derangement.
- Urinalysis may show uric acid crystals.

### ■ Differential Diagnosis

- Volume depletion and prerenal azotemia.
- Nephrotoxic or ischemic acute tubular necrosis (other medications or contrast agents, sepsis, hypotension).
- Obstructive nephropathy secondary to the tumor.
- Rare etiologies of acute renal failure in patients with malignancies: acute interstitial nephritis, glomerulonephritis, and thrombotic microangiopathy.

### ■ Treatment

- Eliminate potential nephrotoxins.
- IV hydration (ideally initiated 48 hours prior to chemotherapy in high-risk patients).
- Induction of alkaline diuresis with IV sodium bicarbonate to maintain urine pH greater than 7.0 should be considered.
- Frequent monitoring of electrolytes.
- Major focus on treatment of hyperuricemia with prophylactic allopurinol and in those patients with very high uric acid levels the use of rasburicase to degrade uric acid.
- Dialysis when conservative and pharmacological treatments are ineffective in correcting metabolic derangements.

### ■ Pearl

*Tumor lysis syndrome creates life-threatening metabolic derangements that require careful monitoring, specific pharmacological therapy, and possibly dialysis.*

Reference

Davidson MB et al: Pathophysiology, clinical consequences, and treatment of tumor lysis syndrome. Am J Med 2004;116:546.

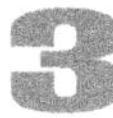

# Chronic Kidney Disease

# Adynamic Bone Disease

- ## Essentials of Diagnosis
  - Adynamic bone disease (ABD) is characterized by reduced synthesis of bone matrix (decreased osteoblastic and osteoclastic activity) and is distinct from osteomalacia (osteoid accumulates due to a lack of osteoblast activity).
  - ABD is one of the most common forms of renal osteodystrophy.
  - While low intact PTH suggests ABD, high iPTH level does not exclude it; thus bone biopsy may be required for diagnosis.
  - High-dose calcium salts for phosphate binding and more frequent and aggressive vitamin D treatment lead to ABD.
  - ABD is more common in the peritoneal dialysis (constant dialysate calcium exposure with suppression of PTH).
  - ABD is seen in association with aging and diabetes, two conditions that predispose to osteoporosis in the general population.
  - It is unknown if ABD is associated with increased morbidity and mortality, but limited data raise these concerns.
  - The main concerns of ABD are related to impaired mineral homeostasis and the increased risk of hip fracture.
  - Age, duration of dialysis, female sex, and diabetes appear to confer an increased risk for fracture.
  - Failure of bone to accrue calcium in ABD may predispose to metastatic calcification and calciphylaxis.

- ## Differential Diagnosis
  - Aluminum-induced bone disease.
  - Osteomalacia, osteitis fibrosa cystica, osteoporosis.
  - Mixed renal osteodystrophy (osteitis fibrosa cystica and ABD).
  - B-2 microglobulin-related bone disease.

- ## Treatment
  - ABD is best treated by increasing bone turnover (increase PTH).
  - Lowering or eliminating doses of calcium-based phosphate binders and vitamin D may increase PTH and bone turnover.
  - Reduced dialysate calcium (1–2 mEq/L) may be beneficial.
  - Agents with potential to increase bone turnover (eg, PTH) are possible candidates for treatment of ABD (experimental).
  - Manipulation of the calcium receptor with calcilytics may help ABD by stimulating PTH release (experimental).

- ## Pearl
*Calcimimetics (cinacalcet), which suppress PTH, but increase the amplitude of PTH cycling may become therapeutic agents for ABD.*

Reference

KDIGO: Clinical practice guideline for the diagnosis, evaluation, prevention, and treatment of chronic kidney disease-mineral and bone disorder. Kidney Int Suppl 2009;(113):S1–130.

## Anemia & Chronic Kidney Disease

- **Essentials of Diagnosis**
  - Normochromic normocytic anemia.
  - Associated with low GFR (CKD Stage III or greater, ie, GFR $<60$ mL/min/1.73 $m^2$); anemia is more common and more severe with GFR less than 30 mL/min/1.73 $m^2$.
  - Etiology is primarily erythropoietin deficiency or resistance.
  - Iron deficiency is common.

- **Differential Diagnosis**
  - Iron deficiency.
  - Gastrointestinal losses.
  - Acute and chronic inflammatory states.
  - Folate and $B_{12}$ deficiencies.
  - Shortened red cell survival/hemolysis.
  - Hemoglobinopathies.

- **Treatment**
  - Treat other causes of anemia.
  - Iron supplementation if deficient (TSAT <20%; Ferritin <100 ng/mL).
  - Exogenous erythropoietin replacement with erythropoiesis-stimulating agents (eg, erythropoietin, darbepoietin).
  - Frequent hemoglobin monitoring (initially every week, then every 2–4 weeks) with erythropoietin replacement.
  - Current guideline for hemoglobin target is approximately 10 g/dL in symptomatic CKD patients but continues to be debated due to concerns over adverse effects (increased stroke risk and progression of cancer).

- **Pearl**

*Iron deficiency and erythropoietin hypo-response/resistance (inflammatory conditions) are leading causes of anemia with CKD; must rule out and treat other secondary causes of anemia.*

**Reference**

Pfeffer MA et al: A trial of darbepoetin alfa in type 2 diabetes and chronic kidney disease. N Engl J Med 2009 Nov19;361(21):2019.

## Atrophic Kidney

### ■ Essentials of Diagnosis
- Small kidney seen on renal ultrasound, computed tomography (CT) scan, or magnetic resonance imaging (MRI).
- Size is usually less than 6 cm in diameter.
- Increased echogenicity on ultrasound and minimal or no uptake of contrast with CT scan or MRI/MRA.
- If congenital renal hypoplasia, hypertrophy of the contralateral kidney is often present (large kidney on ultrasound, CT scan, or MRI).
- Dilated renal pelvis and calyces might be present if renal atrophy is due to chronic ureteral obstruction.

### ■ Differential Diagnosis
- Congenital atrophy (renal hypoplasia).
- Chronic unilateral pyelonephritis.
- Renal artery stenosis (high grade) or renal artery occlusion.
- Chronic unilateral ureteral obstruction from stone, papillary necrosis, blood clot, or malignancy.
- Complete renal infarction from a cardiac embolus, renal artery dissection, or massive cholesterol embolization.

### ■ Treatment
- No specific therapy for the atrophic kidney.
- Control blood pressure if renal artery stenosis is present using medications; sometimes nephrectomy is required.
- Treat infection if chronic pyelonephritis is present and there is evidence of upper tract infection.
- Monitor kidney function more closely if any stage of CKD develops, especially Stage III or greater.

### ■ Pearl
*The presence of an atrophic kidney in patients with underlying vascular disease and hypertension often represents significant renal artery stenosis or occlusion.*

Reference
O'Neill WC: Sonographic evaluation of renal failure. Am J Kidney Dis 2000;35:1021.

## Calciphylaxis

- **Essentials of Diagnosis**
  - More recently known as calcific uremic arteriolopathy (CUA).
  - Occurs in patients with end-stage renal disease (ESRD), advanced chronic kidney disease (CKD stage IV and V), or kidney transplant.
  - Affects up to 5% of dialysis-dependent patients.
  - Rarely occurs in patients without kidney disease (primary hyperparathyroidism, malignancy, chemotherapy, inflammatory bowel disease, connective tissue disease, rapid weight loss).
  - Initial presentation includes very painful, indurated, violaceous plaques, and/or livedo reticularis with ecchymosis.
  - Advanced lesions are severely painful and can be necrotic, ulcerated, and have overlying eschar.
  - Skin biopsy is gold standard for diagnosis but can also precipitate ulcer formation and expansion.
  - Microscopic appearance: circumferential calcium hydroxyapatite deposition in small vessel media (arterioles, venules, and capillaries), intimal proliferation, endovascular fibrosis, and intravascular thrombosis.
  - Risk factors: advanced CKD or dialysis, female sex, diabetes, obesity, elevated phosphate, elevated calcium/phosphate product, hyperparthyroidism.
  - Associations noted with warfarin use in the months prior to diagnosis and subcutaneous injection with nadroparin or insulin.

- **Differential Diagnosis**
  - Warfarin-associated skin necrosis.
  - Clotting disorders including protein C, protein S, and antithrombin III deficiencies.
  - Others: vasculitis, cryoglobulinemia, atheroembolic disease, cellulitis.

- **Treatment**
  - Control calcium and phosphorus levels (low calcium dialysate, non-calcium-containing phosphate binders).
  - Control hyperparathyroidism (parathyroidectomy, cinacalcet).
  - Aggressive wound care and pain control.
  - Hyperbaric oxygen for wound healing.
  - Sodium thiosulfate (cation chelation and antioxidant effects).

- **Pearl**

*Prognosis is poor; up to 80% mortality most often associated with sepsis and wound infection.*

Reference

Rogers NM, Coates PTH: Calcific uraemic arteriolopathy: an update. Curr Opin Nephrol Hypertens 2008;17:629.

## Chronic Kidney Disease (CKD)

- ## Essentials of Diagnosis
  - Estimated CKD prevalence in United States for each stage per the National Health and Nutrition Examination Survey (NHANES) 1999–2004:
    - o  Stage I: 1.8% of total adult US population; Stage II: 3.2%; Stage III: 7.7%; Stage IV: 0.35%; Stage V: 2.4%.
  - CKD is defined by the following criteria per K/DOQI:
    1) Kidney damage for more than 3 months, defined by structural or functional abnormalities of the kidney, with or without decreased GFR, and manifested by either pathological abnormalities; or markers of kidney damage, including abnormalities in the composition of the blood or urine, or imaging abnormalities.
    2) GFR less than 60 mL/min per 1.73 m$^2$ of body surface area for more than 3 months, with or without kidney damage.
  - Annual GFR decline with age is ~1 mL/min after 20 years.
  - CKD classification based on GFR per KDOQI guidelines:
    1) Stage I: GFR greater than 90 mL/min with risk factors.
    2) Stage II: GFR 60–89 mL/min.
    3) Stage III: GFR 30–59 mL/min.
    4) Stage IV: GFR 15–29 mL/min.
    5) Stage V: GFR less than 15 mL/min or dialysis.

- ## Differential Diagnosis
  - Rule out reversible conditions (prolonged AKI) or falsely elevated serum creatinine such as drugs (trimethoprim).

- ## Treatment
  - Identify CKD patients with adequate screening methods.
  - Diagnose comorbid conditions and treat.
  - Prevent progression of CKD with treatment of hypertension, diabetes, proteinuria, acidosis, and bone/mineral diseases.
  - A multidisciplinary approach to care is required.
  - Early referral to nephrology is vital to treat comorbid conditions (anemia, hypertension, metabolic bone disease) and prepare patients mentally and physically for renal replacement therapy and vascular access placement.
  - Review medications regularly to ensure appropriate renal dosing, identify drug interactions, and adverse effects.

- ## Pearl
*Recent evidence suggests that bicarbonate supplementation to correct metabolic acidosis slows the rate of progression to ESRD and improves nutritional status and bone health in CKD patients.*

### Reference

KDIGO: Definition and classification of chronic kidney disease: a position statement from Kidney Disease: Improving global outcomes (KDIGO). Kidney International 2005;67(6):2089–2100.

## Echogenic Kidney

- **Essentials of Diagnosis**
  - Echogenicity is an ultrasound description of renal parenchyma.
  - Ultrasound waves are formed in the transducer, and reflect from tissue interfaces that they pass through back to the transducer.
  - Echogenicity reflects the characteristic ability of a tissue or substance to reflect sound waves and produce echoes.
  - Each tissue type, such as liver, spleen, or kidney, has a particular echogenicity in its normal state.
  - Echogenicity can be used to mean different than the normal echogenicity or compared to another tissue (kidney vs liver).
  - For example, the medulla of the kidney is darker, or less echogenic than the cortex of the kidney on ultrasound.
  - In diseased states, echogenicity of an organ can be altered, either more echogenic (whiter) or less echogenic than usual.
  - The state of echogenicity of the kidneys on ultrasound helps to categorize the type of disease process (along with kidney size, cortical thickness, status of the collecting system, and presence or absence of stones, cysts, or masses).
  - Kidney diseases are more often seen as *echogenic* (ie, more echogenic rather than less echogenic).

- **Differential Diagnosis**
  - Echogenic kidneys (increased echogenicity) are categorized by size (large vs small):
    - Large and echogenic: infiltrative kidney diseases (lymphoma, amyloidosis, Gaucher); diabetes mellitus; cystic kidney diseases; acute interstitial nephritis; acute pyelonephritis; acute glomerulonephrtitis; acute tubular necrosis; HIVAN.
    - Small and echogenic: many forms of CKD (hypertensive nephrosclerosis, renal artery stenosis, chronic pyelonephritis, chronic glomerulonephritis); congenital renal hypoplasia; chronic interstitial nephritis.
  - Rarely, certain diseases are associated with large kidneys with reduced echogenicity such as leukemic renal infiltration and nephrosarca (severe renal edema from nephrotic syndrome).

- **Treatment**
  - Treatment is based on the type of kidney disease diagnosed.

- **Pearl**

*The term "medical renal disease" is nonspecific and generally is used by radiologists to describe "increased echogenicity" of the kidneys with loss of the corticomedullary differentiation (cortex whiter than medulla) normally seen on renal ultrasound.*

Reference

O'Neill WC: Sonographic evaluation of renal failure. Am J Kidney Dis 2000;35:1021.

## End-Stage Renal Disease (ESRD)

- **■ Essentials of Diagnosis**
  - ESRD represents a progression of chronic kidney disease to a GFR less than 10–15 cc/min, which requires renal replacement therapy.
  - As per the USRDS data in 2006, the incidence of ESRD was 360 per million population, a number that is steadily increasing.
  - Symptoms include fatigue, pruritis, weight loss, nausea, loss of appetite, drowsiness, confusion, skin color, and nail changes.
  - The major causes of ESRD are diabetes mellitus and hypertension, although there are several other causes.
  - It is important to identify patients with CKD at a stage that permits time to prepare the patient for dialysis access and/or to refer for preemptive renal transplantation.
  - If hemodialysis is chosen, an AV fistula is the preferred access and should be placed at least 3 months prior to initiation of dialysis.
  - If peritoneal dialysis is the modality of choice, a Tenchkoff catheter is placed approximately 2 weeks prior to dialysis.

- **■ Treatment**
  - It is essential to closely monitor these individuals for timely initiation of dialysis.
  - Other important aspects of management are:
    - ○ Hypertension: volume management and pharmacotherapy.
    - ○ Anemia: ESA, iron supplementation, reduce plebotomy.
    - ○ Renal osteodystrophy: control phosphorous, calcium, and PTH.
  - Vascular access creation and preservation.
  - Appropriate dosing of medications to a GFR less than 10 cc/min.
  - Prevention of infection; appropriate vaccination.
  - Provision of adequate nutrition.

- **■ Pearl**

*There has been recent debate as to the timing of initiation of dialysis. Current evidence suggests that early initiation of dialysis (GFR 10–14 mL/min) is not associated with improvement in survival or clinical outcomes as compared with late initiation (GFR 5–7 mL/min).*

Reference

Cooper BA et al: A randomized, controlled trial of early versus late initiation of dialysis. N Engl J Med 2010;363(7):609.

## Nephrogenic Systemic Fibrosis (NSF)

- **Essentials of Diagnosis**
  - NSF is a systemic fibrosing disorder with its most dominant manifestations in the skin.
  - Edema and erythema develop in the first few weeks.
  - Later, the process progresses with skin changes described as *woody, cobblestoned,* or *peau d' orange.*
  - Symmetrical fibrosis begins in the ankles and wrists with proximal progression in many but not all patients.
  - Pain, dysesthesias, and hyperalgesia are frequently present in affected area.
  - Exposure of patients with advanced, acute, or chronic kidney disease to gadolinium-based contrast agents (GBCA) is thought to be the major cause of NSF.
  - Acute kidney injury (AKI) and CKD with GFR less than 30 mL/min, especially those on dialysis at the time of GBCA exposure are at risk.
  - Deep skin biopsy demonstrates thickened collagen bundles in the dermis with CD 34/Procollagen-I positive spindle cells, and mucin deposition.

- **Differential Diagnoses**
  - Cellulitis in early cases.
  - Scleroderma.
  - Scelromyxedema.
  - Lipodermatosclerosis.
  - Calciphylaxis.
  - Eosinophilic fasciitis.

- **Treatment**
  - There is no effective therapy for NSF; however, resolution or improvement in skin findings has occasionally been noted with recovery from AKI or with kidney transplantation.
  - Physical therapy and optimal pain control are crucial therapies.

- **Pearls**

*Prevention is best achieved by avoiding GBCA exposure in AKI or CKD patients (GFR <30 mL/min), especially those on dialysis. Macrocyclic agents (lowest dose) should be used if the patient requires information that can only be obtained with GBCA MRI/MRA. Hemodialysis following GBCA administration should be considered for those on hemodialysis.*

Reference

Perazella MA: Advanced kidney disease, gadolinium, and nephrogenic systemic fibrosis: the perfect storm. Curr Opin Nephrol Hypertens 2009;18(6):519.

# Renal Osteodystrophy

## ■ Essentials of Diagnosis
- Determine the stage of CKD.
- An increase in serum phosphate and decrease in 1,25 dihydroxyvitamin $D_3$ occurs early (GFR <60 mL/min) in CKD.
- Hypocalcemia occurs later (GFR <20 mL/min) in CKD.
- Secondary hyperparathyroidism (elevated intact PTH) appears at Stage II and continues to worsen with higher CKD stage.
- Patients are at increased risk for hip and vertebral fractures.
- Metabolic bone disorders, which are associated with one or more of the disturbances noted previously, are described:
  ○ Osteitis fibrosa: increased PTH, increased osteoblast and osteoclast activity and number.
  ○ Osteomalacia: 1,25 dihydroxyvitamin $D_3$ deficiency; low bone turnover, unmineralized osteoid.
  ○ Mixed uremic osteodystrophy: features of both of the above bone disorders.
  ○ Adynamic bone disease: reduced bone formation and resorption, low bone turnover.

## ■ Differential Diagnosis
- Osteoporosis.
- K/DOQI practice guidelines for target iPTH levels per CKD stage:
  ○ Stage III CKD: 35–70 pg/mL.
  ○ Stage IV CKD: 70–110 pg/mL.
  ○ Stage V CKD: 150–300 pg/mL.

## ■ Treatment
- Correction of hyperphosphatemia: diet, binders.
- Correction of hypocalcemia: calcium supplementation.
- Correction of acidosis: oral bicarbonate replacement.
- Monitor and correct elevated intact PTH: vitamin D analogues (eg, paracalcitol, calcitriol, doxercalciferol, ergocalciferol), role of cinacalcet is unclear.

## ■ Pearl
*Consider bone biopsy for establishing the type of renal bone disease, since no combination of biochemical parameters is sufficiently accurate.*

References

K/DOQI: Clinical practice guidelines for bone metabolism and disease in chronic kidney disease. Am J Kidney Dis 2003;42(Suppl 3):S1.

KDIGO: Clinical practice guideline for the diagnosis, evaluation, prevention, and treatment of chronic kidney disease—mineral and bone disorder. Kidney Int Suppl 2009;(113):S1–130.

## Uremia

- **Essentials of Diagnosis**
  - Uremic retention of various solutes and toxins.
  - Anemia: fatigue, heart failure, decreased well being.
  - Bleeding tendency: dysfunction of the platelets.
  - Metabolic acidosis: anorexia, poor nutrition.
  - Hyperkalemia: muscular dysfunction and cardiac arrest.
  - Sodium retention: hypertension and heart failure.
  - Metabolic bone disease: secondary hyperparathyroidism, osteomalacia, adynamic bone disease with associated fractures, metastatic calcification, and calcific uremic arteriolopathy.
  - Endocrine abnormalities: reduced insulin clearance and increased insulin secretion; impotence/decreased libido in men and infertility in women; growth impairment in children.
  - Cardiovascular abnormalities: uremic pericarditis, pericardial effusions, coronary and valvular calcification, left ventricular hypertrophy, arrhythmias and atherosclerosis.
  - Malnutrition: anorexia, weight loss, loss of muscle mass, low cholesterol and serum transferrin levels, and hypoalbuminemia.
  - Skin: uremic frost, sallow skin due to urochrome, melanosis.
  - Neurologic system: insomnia, restless legs, asterixis, neuropathy, myoclonus, seizures, carpal tunnel syndrome, and coma.
  - Gastrointestinal: metallic taste, anorexia, gastroparesis,.
  - Others: nail atrophy, pruritus, hiccups, beta 2-microglobulin amyloidosis, increased infection risk.

- **Differential Diagnosis**
  - Anemia: non-CKD related such as infection, inflammation.
  - Encephalopathy: anoxic, toxic, infectious, and metabolic.
  - Pericardial effusion: nonuremic such as infection and cancer.
  - Tremor and myoclonus from nonuremic disorders.
  - Nonuremic metabolic disturbances: hypocalcemia, hyperkalemia, hyperphosphatemia, and metabolic acidosis.

- **Treatment**
  - Hemodialysis (URR >65% and Kt/V >1.2).
  - Peritoneal dialysis (Kt/V target >1.7).
  - Kidney transplant (only definitive cure for uremia).
  - Anemia: erythropoiesis-stimulating agents (ESA), iron.
  - Metabolic bone disease: vitamin $D_3$ analogs, phosphate binders (calcium and non–calcium-based binders).
  - Uremic bleeding: adequate dialysis, desmopressin, cryoprecipitate, tranexamic acid, or conjugated estrogens.
  - Low-potassium, low-phosphate, and low-sodium diets.
  - Protein restriction: 0.8–1.0 g of protein/kg of weight.

- **Pearl**

*Overt signs/symptoms occur when GFR is less than 5–7 mL/min; however, mild signs/symptoms develop earlier.*

Reference

Almeras C, Argiles A: The general picture of uremia. Seminars in Dialysis 2009;22(4):329.

# Uremic Pericarditis

## ■ Essentials of Diagnosis
- Two types of pericarditis are associated with renal failure.
- Uremic pericarditis, which occurs in patients with uremia before or within 8 weeks of initiation of maintenance dialysis.
- Dialysis-associated pericarditis, occurs more than 8 weeks after dialytic therapy is begun (chronic dialysis patient).
- Asymptomatic pericardial effusions (11%–60%) of ESRD patients.
- Pleuritic chest is the most specific symptom.
- Nonspecific symptoms: fever, chills, cough, malaise, headache.
- Large effusions: dyspnea, orthopnea, muffled heart sounds.
- Tachycardia, hypotension, jugular venous distension, Kussmaul sign, elevated pulsus paradoxus, and Ewart sign may indicate impending cardiac tamponade.
- Pericardial friction rub is a specific but insensitive sign.
- EKG may show diffuse ST segment elevation, PR segment depression, low voltage, electrical alternans.
- Echocardiogram is used to monitor effusion size and cardiac tamponade (reflected by right ventricular diastolic collapse).
- Hemorrhage (heparin) can rapidly increase size of the effusion.
- Histology shows organized fibrinous exudate attached to the thickened pericardium with lymphocyte infiltration.

## ■ Differential Diagnosis
- Pericarditis from infection, connective tissue disorders, malignancy, or drugs.
- Constrictive pericarditis.
- Angina/myocardial infarction, aortic dissection, CHF.
- Pulmonary embolism, pneumothorax, GERD.

## ■ Treatment
- Uremic pericarditis is an absolute indication for dialysis.
- Intensive hemodialysis without heparin (daily dialysis for 10–14 days) is initial therapy in hemodynamically stable patients.
- It is less effective for dialysis-associated pericarditis.
- Patients should have serial echocardiograms every 3–5 days.
- Both small (<1 cm echo-free space) and moderate (1–2 cm) effusions should be treated initially with intensive hemodialysis.
- Large (>2 cm) effusions in dialysis-associated pericarditis should be referred immediately for surgery, whereas a trial of intensive dialysis should be employed in uremic pericarditis.
- Surgery is required when pericarditis fails to resolve.
- Pericardial window (open or thoracoscopic) with intra-pericardial glucocorticoid is the surgical procedure of choice.
- Pericardiectomy is effective but has more complications.
- Needle pericardiocentesis has high mortality and recurrence rate.

## ■ Pearl
*Failure to rapidly diagnose uremic pericarditis could result in significant morbidity and increased risk for mortality.*

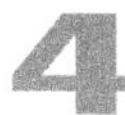# Systemic Diseases Involving the Kidneys

# Diabetic Nephropathy (DN)

## ■ Essentials of Diagnosis
- Diabetes mellitus (DM) is generally present for many years in type-1 patients who develop DN, although type-2 diabetics develop DN within a few years of diagnosis because DM has been present for many years.
- Microalbuminuria (MA) is the earliest clinical manifestation, while some patients develop nephrotic range proteinuria.
- DN is classically divided into the following clinical stages: stage 1, increased GFR; stage 2, MA; stage 3, overt proteinuria; stage 4, decreased GFR, increased proteinuria, hypertension; stage 5, CKD (stage 5) requiring renal replacement therapy.
- Diabetic retinopathy is present in 100% of type 1 diabetes mellitus, while it occurs in only 50–60% of type 2 diabetics.
- DN is frequently complicated by hypertension that requires therapy with multiple medications, including a diuretic.
- Renal biopsy is confirmatory, but is often not necessary as the diagnosis can be made on clinical grounds alone.
- Histologic changes include diffuse glomerular basement membrane thickening, mesangial expansion, Kimmelstiel-Wilson nodules, glomerular sclerosis, vascular disease, and chronic tubulointerstitial disease.

## ■ Differential Diagnosis
- Nondiabetic glomerular diseases especially if proteinuria onset occurs within less than 5 years of diagnosis of DM.
- Hypertensive nephrosclerosis may be difficult to differentiate.

## ■ Treatment
- Strict glycemic control.
- Strict BP control to reduce BP to less than 130/80 mm Hg.
- ACE inhibitor/ARB therapy slow the rate of progression of DN.
- Measures to reduce overall cardiovascular (CV) risk are very important, as DN is an independent risk factor for CV events.

## ■ Pearl
*Failure to reduce proteinuria with ACE-I/ARB could be due to either poor BP control or excessive sodium intake (>5 g/day).*

### Reference
Adler A, Stratton I, Neil H, Yudkin J, Matthews D, Cull C, et al: Association of systolic blood pressure with macrovascular and microvascular complications of type 2 diabetes (UKPDS 36): prospective observational study. BMJ 2000;321(7258):412–419.

## Systemic Lupus Erythematosus and the Kidney

- **Essentials of Diagnosis**
  - Systemic lupus erythematosus (SLE) with renal involvement is an immune-complex glomerulonephritis.
  - Systemic symptoms: arthritis, arthralgia, malar rash, oral ulcers, serositis, alopecia, photosensitivity, cerebritis.
  - Serology of SLE: presence of ANA, anti-dsDNA, anti-Sm, anti-Ra, anti-La, anti-C1q; hypocomplementemia (C2, C3, C4).
  - Urinalysis/microscopy: microscopic hematuria, pyuria, proteinuria/dysmorphic red blood cells, red blood cell casts.
  - Proteinuria can be nonnephrotic or nephritic range.
  - Renal biopsy is recommended for diagnosis, therapy, and prognosis.
  - International Society of Nephrology and Renal Pathology Society Classification of Lupus Nephritis (LN): Class I, minimal mesangial LN; Class II, mesangial proliferative LN; Class III, focal proliferative LN; Class IV, diffuse proliferative LN; Class V, membranous LN; Class VI, advanced sclerosing LN.
  - Immunofluorescence: *full house* (IgG, IgA, IgM, C3, C1q).
  - Electron microscopy: electron-dense deposits.
  - Class I and II LN have better long-term prognosis.
  - Class III and IV are progressive without therapy.
  - 10–30% of proliferative nephritis develops ESRD.
  - A less aggressive lesion may transform to a more aggressive form.

- **Differential Diagnosis**
  - SLE with thrombotic microangiopathy/hemolytic uremic syndrome, anti-cardiolipin syndrome, malignant hypertension.
  - Other glomerulonephritides (post-infectious, IgA nephropathy).

- **Treatment**
  - Immunosuppression for class III, IV, or V with features of class III or IV.
  - Induction therapy: steroids and cyclophosphamide or mycophenolate mofetil (MMF).
  - Maintenance therapy: azathioprine or MMF; low-dose steroids.

- **Pearl**

*LN typically occurs within the first few years of SLE diagnosis and adds significant morbidity and mortality.*

Reference

Weening JJ, D'Agati VD, Schwartz MM, et al: The classification of glomerulonephritis in systemic lupus erythematosus revisited. J Am Soc Nephrol 2004;15:241–250.

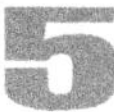

# Glomerular Disorders

## Nephrotic Syndrome

- **Essentials of Diagnosis**
  - Defined as severe proteinuria (typically >3 g of albuminuria per day), edema, and hypoalbuminemia.
  - Generally accompanied by hyperlipidemia and a prothrombotic state.
  - Other complications may include protein malnutrition, acute renal failure, volume depletion.
  - Urine microscopy may show lipiduria including fatty casts, free fat droplets, and oval fat bodies (seen as maltese crosses under polarized light).
  - The presence of nephrotic syndrome implies an underlying glomerular disease.
  - Renal biopsy is required to determine the etiology and subsequent treatment of nephrotic syndrome.
  - Further tests include renal ultrasound, serum complement levels, serum and urine protein immunofixation, hepatitis, and other serological tests to distinguish the causes noted below.

- **Differential Diagnosis**
  - Primary glomerular diseases: membranous nephropathy (MN), minimal change disease (MCD), focal segmental glomerulosclerosis, idiopathic type I MPGN and dense deposit disease, IgA nephropathy.
  - Secondary glomerular diseases: diabetic glomerulosclerosis; lupus nephritis; infection associated (eg, hepatitis C-associated MPGN, HIVAN), drug associated (eg, NSAID-associated MCD), cancer associated (eg, Hodgkin lymphoma-associated MCD), carcinoma-associated MN, amyloidosis and light chain deposition disease, fibrillary glomerulopathy, or immunotactoid glomerulopathy.

- **Treatment**
  - Treatment of the glomerular disease depends on the etiology.
  - ACE inhibitors or ARBs are recommended for blood pressure control and to reduce proteinuria.
  - Oral salt restriction and loop diuretics are used for edema.
  - HMG CoA inhibitors may be needed to treat hyperlipidemia.
  - Anticoagulation may be necessary if patients develop thromboembolism.

- **Pearl**

*All patients presenting with edema or unexplained weight gain should be tested for albuminuria.*

Reference

Orth S, Ritz E: The nephrotic syndrome. N Engl J Med 1998;338(17):1202.

## Minimal Change Disease (MCD)

- **Essentials of Diagnosis**
  - Disease onset often in childhood and the incidence drops with rising age.
  - Accounts for roughly 50–90% of nephrotic syndrome in children and 10–15% of primary nephrotic syndrome in adults.
  - Presents with sudden onset of nephrotic syndrome, including heavy proteinuria, hypoalbuminemia, edema, and hyperlipidemia.
  - Rarely accompanied by hypertension.
  - Occasionally presents with acute renal failure.
  - Urine microscopy shows oval fat bodies and fatty casts.
  - Serum complement levels are normal and serological tests are negative for autoantibodies.
  - Diagnosis is made presumptively in children based on the high prevalence, and by renal biopsy in adults.
  - Light microscopy shows minimal cellularity in glomeruli and normal tubular and interstitial structure; immunofluorescence is negative.
  - Electron microscopy shows effacement of epithelial foot processes.
  - Causes of secondary MCD include Hodgkin lymphoma, hypersensitivity to drugs (eg, NSAID, penicillin), and insect stings.

- **Differential Diagnosis**
  - Focal segmental glomerulosclerosis.
  - Membranous nephropathy.
  - Amyloidosis and light chain deposition disease.
  - Fibrillary or immunotactoid glomerulonephropathy.

- **Treatment**
  - Corticosteroid is first-line therapy in children and adults.
  - Steroid-resistant subtypes may require alternative immunomodulating therapy including cyclophosphamide, cyclosporine, tacrolimus, or mycophenolate mofetil.
  - Steroid-dependent or frequent-relapsing types may require low-dose prednisone for a longer duration or repeat kidney biopsy to evaluate any change in pathology.

- **Pearl**

*MCD should be included in the differential diagnosis in any patient presenting with sudden onset of severe nephrotic syndrome, even elderly patients.*

Reference

Mathieson PW: Minimal change nephropathy and focal segmental glomerulosclerosis. Semin Immunopathol 2007;29:415.

# IgM Nephropathy

## ■ Essentials of Diagnosis
- An idiopathic proteinuric glomerular disease with mesangial hypercellularity and diffuse IgM deposits seen on immunofluorescence.
- Electron microscopy may show mesangial deposits.
- May represent a variant of minimal change disease or focal segmental glomerulosclerosis as opposed to being a separate entity. IgM deposits have been described with equal frequency in patients with minimal change disease, focal segmental glomerulosclerosis, and mesangial proliferative glomerulonephritis.
- Presents with proteinuria (often nephrotic range), microscopic hematuria, and hypertension.
- Age of onset varies from young children to elderly over 70 years.
- Approximately one-third of patients develop end-stage renal disease at up to 15 years post-diagnosis.
- Less likely to respond to steroids than minimal change disease.

## ■ Differential Diagnosis
- Minimal change disease.
- Focal and segmental glomerulosclerosis.
- Mesangial proliferative glomerulonephritis.

## ■ Treatment
- Steroids, though response rates are no better than 50%.
- Cyclophosphamide tends to have low response rates and in those who do go into remission relapses are common.
- Cyclosporine has been shown to be effective in children.

## ■ Pearl
*IgM nephropathy is often described as a separate entity, but it may be a variant of minimal change disease, focal and segmental glomerulosclerosis. The presence of mesangial proliferation portends a poor response to steroids.*

### Reference
Myllymaki J S et al: IgM nephropathy: clinical picture and long-term prognosis. Am J Kid Dis 2003;41:343.

# Focal Segmental Glomerulosclerosis (FSGS)

## ■ Essentials of Diagnosis
- Cause of 10–20% of nephrotic syndrome, with a rising incidence among the African Americans.
- Presents with variable degree of proteinuria, hypertension, microscopic hematuria, and decreased glomerular filtrate rate.
- Patients also may have signs of tubulointerstitial injury.
- Primary (idiopathic) FSGS is a diffuse podocyte disease that typically presents with severe proteinuria.
- Secondary FSGS causes patchy podocyte damage and often manifests with subnephrotic proteinuria; causes include genetic mutations of podocyte proteins, HIV, parovirus B19, pamidronate, reduced nephron mass, and hyperfiltration from vesico-ureteral reflux nephropathy, obesity, and sickle cell disease.
- Kidney biopsy demonstrates areas of glomerular scarring in parts of glomerular tufts on light microscopy and effacement of podocytes on electron microscopy; immunofluorescence is negative.
- Five histological variants of FSGS include: tip lesion, collapsing, cellular, perihilar, and not-otherwise-specified. Tip lesion is most responsive and collapsing variety is least responsive to treatment.

## ■ Differential Diagnosis
- Minimal change disease.
- Membranous nephropathy.
- Diabetic nephropathy.
- Amyloidosis.
- IgA nephropathy.
- Membranoproliferative glomerulonephritis.

## ■ Treatment
- First-line therapy for idiopathic FSGS is steroid therapy. Second-line therapy includes other cytotoxic agents such as cyclosporine, cyclophosphamide. Mycophenolate mofetil and tacrolimus. These are being studied in multicenter trial.
- Treatment of secondary FSGS is directed at the underlying cause, such as antiretroviral therapy for HIV-associated FSGS.
- Angiotensin converting enzyme (ACE) inhibitors or angiotensin receptor blockers (ARB) are particularly effective in secondary forms with reduced renal mass.
- Non-immunosuppressive therapy such as strict blood pressure control and lipid control are recommended in all cases.

## ■ Pearl
*Strong association with mutations in the gene encoding APOL1 in patients of African ancestry.*

Reference
Mathieson PW: Minimal change nephropathy and focal segmental glomerulosclerosis. Semin Immunopathol 2007;29:415.

## Membranous Nephropathy (MN)

- **Essentials of Diagnosis**
  - Most common cause of idiopathic nephrotic syndrome in adults.
  - Presents with nephrotic syndrome (heavy proteinuria, edema, and hypoalbuminemia), usually with preserved kidney function. Uncommonly, some may have sub-nephrotic proteinuria or impaired renal function.
  - Urine microscopy may be bland or show oval fat bodies and fatty casts. Microscopic hematuria may be present.
  - Secondary MN may be associated with lupus, hepatitis B, NSAIDs, gold, penicillamine, mercury, and solid-organ carcinomas.
  - Kidney biopsy light microscopy shows normal glomerular basement membrane (GBM) in early stages. Later, the GBM is diffusely thickened with spikes on silver methenamine stains.
  - Intense, fine granular deposits of IgG (especially IgG4) and C3 are present on the glomerular capillary walls on immunofluorescence. Electron microscopy shows subepithelial immune deposits, GBM expansion between the deposits and effacement of the overlying podocyte foot processes.
  - Serum complement levels are normal in primary MN.
  - Patients with severe nephrotic syndrome are at risk for renal vein and deep vein thrombosis and pulmonary embolism.

- **Differential Diagnosis**
  - FSGS.
  - Minimal change disease.
  - MPGN.
  - Diabetic nephropathy.
  - Amyloidosis.

- **Treatment**
  - Nearly 20–30% of idiopathic MN enters remission spontaneously.
  - Low-grade proteinuria may be treated with ACE inhibitors and statins and diuretics if necessary.
  - High-grade proteinuria may need to be treatment with cyclophosphamide and steroids, cyclosporine, or rituximab.
  - Treatment of secondary MN should be focused on removing the offending agent or treatment of the underlying cause.
  - Those with thromboembolic complications or persistent high-grade proteinuria require long-term anticoagulation.

- **Pearl**

*A high proportion of patients with primary MN have circulating anti-phospholipase A2 receptor antibodies.*

Reference

Beck L: Recent advances in membranous nephropathy. Nephrol Round 2009;7(7).

## Idiopathic Nodular Glomerulosclerosis

- **Essentials of Diagnosis**
  - Typically elderly patient with history of long-standing hypertension and smoking.
  - Association with smoking led to recommendation that it be named "smoking-associated nodular glomerulosclerosis".
  - Often have hyperlipidemia and vascular disease but no evidence of diabetes mellitus.
  - Present with renal failure, proteinuria.
  - 20% of patients have nephrotic syndrome.
  - Biopsy resembles nodular diabetic glomerulosclerosis (Kimmelstiel-Wilson nephropathy) with diffuse and nodular mesangial sclerosis, thickening of GBM, and arteriolosclerosis.
  - Smoking likely leads to development of nodular glomerulosclerosis by inducing oxidative stress, angiogenesis, and altered intrarenal hemodynamics.
  - Smoking may also lead to the formation of advanced glycation end products.

- **Differential Diagnosis**
  - Diabetic nephropathy.
  - Amyloidosis.
  - Light and heavy chain deposition disease.
  - Fibrillary or immunotactoid glomerulonephritis.
  - Membranoproliferative glomerulonephritis.
  - Takayasu arteritis.

- **Treatment**
  - Smoking cessation.
  - ACE-inhibitors or angiotensin receptor blockers.
  - Progression to ESRD common.

- **Pearl**

*Occurs in smokers and resembles diabetic nephropathy on biopsy though patients do not have glucose intolerance.*

**Reference**

Markowitz GS et al: Idiopathic nodular glomerulosclerosis is a distinct clinico-pathologic entity linked to hypertension and smoking. Hum Pathol 2002;33:826.

# C1q Nephropathy

## ■ Essentials of Diagnosis
- A rare proteinuric disease characterized by mesangial proliferation and prominent C1q deposits on immunofluorescence.
- C1q staining is usually accompanied by staining for IgG, IgM, and C3.
- Light microscopic findings vary from no lesion to focal segmental sclerosing lesions to proliferative glomerulonephritis.
- Renal manifestations resemble lupus nephritis but there is no clinical or serological evidence of SLE.
- Patients are usually between ages 15 and 30 years.
- Black to white ratio 5:1 and males to females 1.8:1.
- All patients have proteinuria (nephrotic range in more than half).
- Edema, hypertension, hematuria, and CKD are common features.
- Patients with features of FSGS on light microscopy are more likely to have nephrotic range proteinuria and progress to ESRD.

## ■ Differential Diagnosis
- Minimal change disease.
- Focal and segmental glomerulosclerosis.
- Mesangial proliferative glomerulonephritis.

## ■ Treatment
- Treatment is guided by the clinical and histological features.
- Patients with subnephrotic proteinuria and a minimal change lesion may require only ACE inhibitor or ARB treatment.
- Steroids are typically initiated first for those with nephrotic syndrome, followed by cyclosporine or cyclophosphamide for steroid-resistant or -dependent patients.
- Patients with nephrotic syndrome, particularly with FSGS features are more resistant to steroids and show higher incidences of progression to ESRD.

## ■ Pearl
*C1q nephropathy may be a subgroup of other glomerular diseases such as minimal change disease, focal segmental glomerulosclerosis, or proliferative glomerulonephritis, and treatment should be directed to the underlying disease suggested on light microscopy.*

Reference

Vizjak, A et al: Pathology, clinical presentations, and outcomes of C1q nephropathy. J Am Soc Nephrology 2008;19:2237.

## HIV-Associated Nephropathy (HIVAN)

- **Essentials of Diagnosis**
  - Renal failure and massive proteinuria though peripheral edema is often absent.
  - Usually normotensive.
  - More common in African American patients; associated with APOL1 mutations.
  - Rapid progression to ESRD.
  - Third most common cause of ESRD in the USA among African American adult males (between the ages of 20–64 years).
  - Most patients have low CD4 counts and have been HIV seropositive for several years, though there have been reports in all stages of infection including acute seroconversion.
  - Renal ultrasound shows large, echogenic kidneys.
  - Biopsy shows collapsing FSGS with tubular microcystic dilatation with proteinaceous casts. Electron microscopy shows tubuloreticular inclusions in the glomerular endothelial cells.

- **Differential Diagnosis**
  - Idiopathic collapsing glomerulopathy.
  - Other causes of adult-onset nephrotic syndrome.
  - Other glomerular diseases have been described in HIV including an HIV-associated immune complex disease and HIV-associated thrombotic microangiopathy.
  - IgA nephropathy, postinfectious glomerulonephritis, and MPGN occur at increased frequencies in HIV.
  - Membranoproliferative glomerulonephritis and membranous nephropathy may occur with hepatitis C and/ or hepatitis B coinfection.
  - Nephrotoxicity due to medications.

- **Treatment**
  - Anti-retroviral therapy of HIV-infected patients has reduced the incidence of HIVAN and may result in stabilization of renal function and sometimes in clinical and pathological improvement.
  - Secondary treatment measures including ACE-inhibition or angiotensin receptor blockers and cholesterol-lowering therapy.

- **Pearl**

*Renal transplantation has become a feasible option for patients with HIVAN who develop ESRD.*

Reference

Weiner NJ et al: The HIV-associated renal diseases: current insight into pathogenesis and treatment. Kid Int 2003;63:1618.

# Renal Vein Thrombosis (RVT)

## ■ Essentials of Diagnosis
- Usually occurs in the setting of a hypercoagulable state (nephrotic syndrome, clotting disorders such deficiencies in protein C, protein S, and antithrombin III, active tumors, and anti-phospholipid antibody syndrome).
- Other causes include interventions on the renal vein, trauma, retroperitoneal fibrosis, and acute vascular rejection post transplant.
- Membranous nephropathy is the most common cause of nephrotic syndrome that leads to renal vein thrombosis (5–62% of cases).
- Acute thrombosis presents with loin pain and hematuria, and less commonly, fever, worsening of proteinuria, and acute renal failure if bilateral or in a single kidney.
- Chronic thrombosis is often asymptomatic and may be discovered incidentally in a patient with a pulmonary embolism.
- Labs may reveal an elevated LDH and renal ultrasound shows an increase in kidney size.
- Renal venography is the gold standard for diagnosis; other options include spiral computed tomography with contrast, magnetic resonance imaging, and Doppler ultrasonography.
- No proven benefit to routine screening in patients with nephrotic syndrome.

## ■ Differential Diagnosis
- Renal infarct.
- Loin pain hematuria syndrome.
- Pyelonephritis.
- Nephrolithiasis.

## ■ Treatment
- Nephrotic patients with serum albumin less than 2 g/dL and proteinuria greater than 5 g may warrant prophylaxis if other risk factors for embolic events are present.
- Documented RVT is treated with anticoagulation for at least 6 months, with possible extension if massive proteinuria persists.
- Local thrombolytic therapy with thrombectomy has been used with acute RVT and acute kidney injury.
- IVC filter for patients who cannot be anticoagulated.
- Treatment of underlying nephrotic syndrome or malignancy.

## ■ Pearl
*Patients found to have RVT in the absence of nephrotic syndrome should be screened for a clotting disorder or malignancy.*

Reference

Rabelink TJ et al: Thrombosis and hemostasis in renal disease. Kidney Int 1994; 46:287.

## Post-streptococcal Glomerulonephritis (PSGN)

- **Essentials of Diagnosis**
  - Common cause of acute nephritis worldwide; immune complex deposition induced by specific "nephritogenic" strains of group A β-hemolytic streptococcus.
  - Nephritis-associated plasmin receptor and streptococcal pyrogenic exotoxin B are antigens that activate the alternative complement pathway and are actively being investigated as primary causes of PSGN.
  - More common in children and in developing countries.
  - Occurs 1–3 weeks after a group A streptococcal pharyngitis or up to 6 weeks after a group A streptococcal skin infection.
  - "Nephritic syndrome" – oliguria with dark urine (hematuria), edema, hypertension, and AKI.
  - RBCs and RBC casts with subnephrotic proteinuria.
  - C3 and CH50 are depressed in the first 2 weeks with normal C4. Streptozyme test is highly sensitive in PSGN.
  - Light microscopy shows diffuse proliferative nephritis and immunofluorescence reveals granular C3 and IgG deposition in a mesangial, capillary wall ("garland"), or diffuse ("starry sky") pattern. Electron microscopy shows classic subepithelial "humps" (dome-shaped deposits under effaced epithelium).

- **Differential Diagnosis**
  - Membranoproliferative glomerulonephritis.
  - IgA nephropathy.
  - Lupus nephritis.
  - Post infectious glomerulonephritis due to nongroup A streptococci.

- **Treatment**
  - Conservative therapy with antihypertensives, diuretics, and occasionally, dialysis.
  - Antibiotics for active infection, though most infections have typically resolved at presentation.
  - Prognosis excellent with resolution of hypocomplementemia and AKI at 3–4 weeks.
  - Hematuria and proteinuria may take several weeks to years to resolve.
  - Sporadic cases in adults may not resolve completely.

- **Pearl**

*Persistent renal dysfunction and hypocomplementemia at 2–4 weeks may require renal biopsy and entertainment of alternate diagnoses, despite recent Group A strep infection.*

Reference

Kanjanabuch T, et al: An update of acute postinfectious glomerulonephritis worldwide. Nature Rev Nephrol 2009;5:259.

# Post-infectious Glomerulonephritis

## ■ Essentials of Diagnosis
- Immunologic response of the kidneys that follows a nonrenal infection, most commonly streptococci.
- Occurs primarily in children and young adults in developing countries with a male predominance.
- Infective endocarditis and other endovascular infections are a common cause among intravenous drug abusers.
- Alcoholism, malnutrition, and diabetes increase risk.
- Three major patterns of clinical manifestations include:
  (a) Acute nephritic syndrome (proteinuria, hematuria, edema, HTN and AKI 10–20 days following a pharyngitic or skin infection).
  (b) Rapidly progressive glomerulonephritis.
  (c) Subclinical or asymptomatic glomerulonephritis (microscopic hematuria, pyuria, subnephrotic proteinuria).
- Broad range of offending organisms including streptococci, staphylococci and gram negative bacteria, mycobacteria, fungi, viruses (hepatitis, HIV), and parasites.
- Patholologic patterns seen include:
  Endocapillary exudative glomerulonephritis (Group A streptococci).
  Endocapillary plus extracapillary (crescentic GN).
  Membranoproliferative glomerulonephritis (hepatitis C, shunt nephritis, bacterial endocarditis, or visceral abscesses).
- Labs may show hypocomplementemia and streptozyme test may be positive in patients with group A β-hemolytic streptococcus.

## ■ Differential Diagnosis
- IgA nephropathy.
- Lupus nephritis.
- Hemolytic uremic syndrome.

## ■ Treatment
- Eradication of offending infection with appropriate antimicrobials and/or surgical drainage or excision.
- Supportive therapy with antihypertensives, diuretics, and dialysis if necessary until recovery of renal function.
- Corticosteroids or cytotoxic agents may have a role in patients who fail to improve after eradication of the causative agent, but no randomized trials have proven their efficacy.

## ■ Pearl
*An infectious cause should be sought in all patients with otherwise unexplained acute immune complex glomerulonephritis.*

Reference

Kanjanabuch T, et al: An update of acute postinfectious glomerulonephritis worldwide. Nature Rev Nephrol 2009;5:259.

## Shunt Nephritis

- **Essentials of Diagnosis**
  - Immune complex glomerulonephritis associated with chronic infection of a ventriculoatrial shunt.
  - Clinical features include renal insufficiency of variable severity, low-grade fever, hematuria, proteinuria (usually subnephrotic), hypertension, and anemia.
  - Onset of symptoms may occur weeks to years after shunt surgery or revision.
  - Lab tests reveal hypocomplementemia and occasionally, positive cryoglobulins and anti-nuclear antibodies.
  - Kidney biopsy reveals membranoproliferative glomerulonephritis type I with granular deposits of IgG, IgM, and C3 on immuno-fluorescence and subendothelial and mesangial deposits on electron microscopy.
  - Staphylococcus epidermidis (70–75%) and propionibacterium acnes (7%) are the organisms most commonly cultured from the blood or shunt.

- **Differential Diagnosis**
  - Idiopathic MPGN type I.
  - MPGN type I from other chronic infections (eg, hepatitis C and cryoglobulinemia, infective endocarditis), nephritis, or lymphoma.

- **Treatment**
  - Shunt removal.
  - Intravenous and occasionally intra-ventricular antibiotics.
  - Transient external drainage and future conversion to a ventriculoperitoneal shunt in those that require permanent CSF drainage.
  - Prognosis for improvement of proteinuria and renal function is usually good if shunt is removed in a timely fashion, but may take several months.

- **Pearl**

*Most reported cases of shunt nephritis have occurred in patients with ventriculoatrial shunts, and the increased use of ventriculoperitoneal shunts may explain the decreasing incidence over the past 10 years (17 reported cases).*

Reference

Kiryluk K et al: A young man with Proprionibacterium acnes-induced shunt nephritis. Kidney Int 2008;73,1434.

## Membranoproliferative Glomerulonephritis (MPGN)

- ■ **Essentials of Diagnosis**
  - MPGN is a pattern of glomerular histopathology characterized by glomerular hypercellularity and reduplication of the glomerular basement membrane (GBM) – "tram tracking".
  - MPGN presents with variable amounts of proteinuria, hematuria, hypertension, and mixed nephritic-nephrotic features; some may present with rapidly progressive GN.
  - Types I and III MPGN are immune complex diseases characterized by subendothelial and mesangial deposits on electron microscopy; both have IgG and C3 deposits and sometimes IgM on immunofluorescence; type III also has subepithelial immune deposits.
  - Type I/III may be idiopathic but may be secondary to hepatitis C, infective endocarditis, lupus or B cell lymphoma.
  - Serum C3 and C4 are reduced (C4 often markedly so) in type I/III and tests for hepatitis C, lupus, cryoglobulinemia, and rheumatoid factor may be positive.
  - Dense deposit disease (DDD; formerly Type II MPGN) is most often idiopathic, occurs in young adults, and is characterized by electron-dense bands in the GBM, mesangium, and tubular basement membranes that stain for C3 but not IgG; it may be associated with partial lipodystrophy and results from abnormalities of alternative complement pathway regulation; often associated with positive serology for C3 nephritic factor.
  - DDD frequently progresses to end-stage renal disease and recurs after transplantation.

- ■ **Differential Diagnosis**
  - Thrombotic microangiopathies.
  - Lupus nephritis.
  - Immunoglobulin deposition diseases.
  - Immunotactoid nephropathy.

- ■ **Treatment**
  - Idiopathic MPGN may be treated with corticosteroids but remission is rare. RPGN may be halted with pulse steroid.
  - Secondary MPGN associated with hepatitis C is treated with interferon and ribavirin.
  - Treatment of DDD is unsatisfactory; experimental therapies include plasma exchange and Rituximab.

- ■ **Pearl**

*Diagnosis of MPGN should be evaluated for systemic infections or liver disease.*

Reference

Rennke HG: Secondary membranoproliferative glomerulonephritis (Nephrology Forum). Kid Int 1995;47:643.

## Hepatitis C Virus-Associated Nephropathy

- **Essentials of Diagnosis**
  - Hepatitis C has been associated with type I membranoproliferative glomerulonephritis (MPGN) with or without cryoglobulinemia, and less commonly membranous nephropathy, focal segmental glomerulosclerosis, and thrombotic microangiopathy. The most prominent form of hepatitis C nephropathy is type I MPGN.
  - Patients may also have extrarenal features of mixed cryoglobulinemia.
  - Renal manifestations include proteinuria (nephrotic or subnephrotic), microscopic hematuria, and decreased kidney function.
  - Laboratory studies show positive hepatitis C antibodies, HCV RNA viral load, positive rheumatoid factor, low level of complement C4 and C3, and 50–70% may have positive cryoglobulin levels (cryocrit usually <3%); liver function and enzymes may be abnormal.
  - Kidney biopsy shows immune complex deposition in subendothelial space, mesangial hypercellularity, splitting of glomerular basement membrane, lobular architecture. Glomerular capillaries may also have marked inflammatory cell infiltrates with both mononuclear cells and polymorphonuclear leukocytes.

- **Differential Diagnosis**
  - Idiopathic MPGN.
  - Thrombotic microangiopathy.
  - Other post-infectious glomerulonephritis.
  - Small vessel vasculitis.
  - Lupus nephritis.

- **Treatment**
  - Anti-HCV therapy: includes peg-interferon and ribavirin.
  - Immunosuppressive therapy: plasma exchange, corticosteroids, cyclophosphamide. However, hepatitis C viral titers may increase with immunosuppression.
  - Anti-CD20 therapy (rituximab) has been reported beneficial in selected cases.

- **Pearl**

*Hepatitis C nephropathy often manifests as type I MPGN with or without mixed cryoglobulinemia.*

Reference

Meyers C et al: Hepatitis C and renal disease: an update. Am J Kid Dis 2003;42(4):631.

## Cryoglobulinemic Glomerulonephritis

■ Essentials of Diagnosis
- Cryoglobulins are circulating immunoglobulins (Ig) that precipitate upon cooling. There are three types.
- Type I: High levels of monoclonal Ig, mostly IgM or IgG, often due to Waldenstrom macroglobulinemia or multiple myeloma.
- Type II: Moderate levels of monoclonal IgM rheumatoid factor against polyclonal IgG, often associated with hepatitis C and sometimes with B cell lymphoma/leukemia..
- Type III: Low levels of polyclonal IgG or IgM directed against polyclonal IgG, often associated with infectious or autoimmune diseases.
- Mixed cryoglobulinemia (most often Type II) manifests with weakness, palpable purpura, arthralgia, neuropathy, glomerulonephritis, and vasculitis of other organs including GI tract, heart, lungs, and central nervous system.
- Renal manifestation: slow and indolent course, mixed nephritic-nephrotic features, or may present with RPGN. Renal biopsy shows type I MPGN.
- Serology: positive serum cryoglobulins; low complement C4 and mildly or moderately decreased C3 levels; positive rheumatoid factor; hepatitis C antibodies and PCR may be positive.
- Type I cryoglobulinemia manifests with hyperviscosity, Raynaud phenomenon, and livedo reticularis.

■ Differential Diagnosis
- Other small vessel vasculitis.

■ Treatment
- Mild asymptomatic disease: conservative therapy; cold avoidance.
- Symptomatic disease: target underlying lymphoproliferative disease or associated hepatitis C.
- Patients with active nephritis may need plasmapheresis, high-dose steroids, and cytotoxic agents.

■ Pearl

*Mixed cryoglobulinema is often associated with chronic hepatitis C infection and type I MPGN.*

Reference

Jennette JC, Falk R: Small vessel vasculitis. N Engl J Med 1997;337(21):1512.

## IgA Nephropathy

### Essentials of Diagnosis

- More common in males than in females.
- Most common form of acute and chronic glomerulonephritis in Asians and Caucasians.
- Can present as macroscopic hematuria, asymptomatic hematuria with or without proteinuria, nephrotic syndrome, acute renal failure (rare), and chronic kidney disease (CKD).
- Episodic macroscopic hematuria accompanied by flank pain is often seen in the second and third decades of life, generally precipitated by mucosal infections.
- Diagnosis is by kidney biopsy.
- Pathology typically shows mesangial hypercellularity on light microscopy. Diffuse mesangial deposits of IgA are pathognomonic often accompanied by C3. In acute renal failure, necrotizing glomerulonephritis with crescent formation or tubular occlusion by red blood cells may be seen. Electron microscopy reveals electron-dense deposits corresponding to mesangial IgA..
- Serum IgA levels may be elevated but are not sensitive or specific for the diagnosis.
- Serum complement levels are normal but an elevated serum IgA/C3 ratio is seen in more severe cases.
- The IgA1 deposits are abnormally glycosylated and IgG anti-IgA1 antibodies are present in some cases.
- Persistent proteinuria, hypertension, and elevated creatinine at baseline are poor prognostic indictors for the development of CKD.

### Differential Diagnosis

- Thin-basement membrane disease.
- Hereditary nephritis.
- Henoch-Schönlein purpura.
- Post-streptococcal glomerulonephritis.
- Anti-GBM disease.
- ANCA-associated renal vasculitis.
- Lupus nephritis.
- Nonglomerular causes of hematuria such as stones, medullary sponge kidney, and neoplasia.

### Treatment

- Recurrent macroscopic or isolated microscopic hematuria requires only supportive therapy.
- ACE inhibitor or ARB to reduce proteinuria.
- Tight control of blood pressure.
- Persistent proteinuria greater than 1 g/24 hour and preserved renal function is an indication for a 6-month course of prednisone.
- Hematuria with acute renal failure requires pulse methylprednisolone.
- Use of fish oil up to 12 g/d is controversial.

### Reference

Donadio J, Grande J. Medical Progress: IgA Nephropathy; 2002:347:738–748.

# Henoch-Schönlein Nephropathy (HSN)

- **Essentials of Diagnosis**
  - Henoch-Schönlein purpura (HSP) is a small vessel vasculitis with IgA deposition in the skin, joints, gastrointestinal tract, and kidney.
  - Often presents in childhood, but can occur at any age; often preceded by an infection; no specific antigen identified.
  - Extrarenal manifestations include palpable purpura especially on extensor surfaces of lower limbs and buttocks, polyarthralgia, abdominal pain, vomiting, hematochezia, or melena.
  - HSN is often transient; it typically occurs days to weeks after, but may precede, the onset of systemic symptoms.
  - HSN mostly presents with microscopic hematuria, proteinuria, and active sediment but sometimes as nephrotic syndrome or RPGN.
  - As in IgA nephropathy (IgAN), light microscopy shows mesangial proliferation but may show focal necrotizing lesions with crescents in severe cases. Mesangial desposits of IgA and/or IgG, and C3 but not C4 are found on immunofluorescence. Electron microscopy shows mesangial and sometimes capillary loop deposits.
  - Serological tests are negative except for an elevated IgA/C3 ratio in some cases.
  - As in IgAN, the IgA1 deposits are abnormally glycosylated and IgG anti-IgA1 antibodies are present in some cases.
  - Poorer prognosis in adults and among those with persistent proteinuria, hypertension, and elevated creatinine at baseline.

- **Differential Diagnosis**
  - Other small vessel vasculitis.
  - Lupus nephritis.
  - IgA monoclonal gammopathy.

- **Treatment**
  - Mild HSN often resolves spontaneously and requires only supportive measures, ACE inhibitor, or ARB to reduce proteinuria and tight control of blood pressure.
  - Persistent proteinuria greater than 1 g/24 hour and preserved renal function is an indication for a 6-month course of prednisone.

- **Pearl**

*HSN is differentiated from IgAN by the extrarenal manifestations.*

Reference

Davin JC et al: What is the difference between IgA nephropathy and Henoch-Schönlein purpura nephritis. Kidney Int 2001;59:823.

# Lupus Nephritis (LN)

## ■ Essentials of Diagnosis

- Nephritis is present among 20–40% of patients with systemic lupus erythematosus.
- The disease is more prevalent and more severe among patients of African ancestry and among lower socio-economic groups.
- World Health Organization (WHO) classification: normal (class I); mesangial proliferation (class II); focal proliferation (class III); diffuse proliferation (class IV); membranous nephropathy (class V); advanced sclerosing type (class VI).
- Class III and class IV are considered a spectrum of inflammatory glomerular disease: class III has less than 50% of proliferative and necrotizing glomeruli involvement and class IV greater than 50%. Patients present with nephritic features and decreased kidney function.
- Class V resembles idiopathic membranous nephropathy and often presents with nephrotic syndrome.
- Patients with class III or IV LN usually have decreased C3 and C4 levels and an elevated anti-dsDNA level. Patients with class V may have normal complement levels, ANA, and anti-dsDNA.

## ■ Differential Diagnosis

- Class III/IV LN: IgA nephropathy, post-strep GN, MPGN, RPGN.
- Class V LN: membranous nephropathy, FSGS, or MPGN.
- Other types of lupus involvement include interstitial nephritis, thrombotic microangiopathy and/or anti-phospholipid antibody syndrome, or NSAID-induced kidney disease.

## ■ Treatment

- Strict blood pressure control; ACE inhibitors or ARBs to reduce proteinuria, and statins for hypelipidemia in all cases.
- Severe class III and IV LN induction therapy: monthly IV cyclophosphamide or daily oral mycophenolate mofetil (MMF) and steroid; maintain remission with MMF or azathioprine.
- Various treatments have been proposed for class V LN including cyclophosphamide, cyclosporine, MMF, and prednisone.

## ■ Pearl

*LN tends to be more severe and prevalent among African American lupus patients.*

Reference

Lightstone L: Lupus nephritis: where are we now? Curr Opin Rheumatol 2010;22:252.

# Rapidly Progressive Glomerulonephritis

## ■ Essentials of Diagnosis

- Rapid decline in renal function over weeks to months with extensive (>50%) crescent formation on renal biopsy.
- Extent of crescent formation correlates with the degree of renal failure and can predict response to treatment.
- Four types of crescentic GN based on immunofluorecence:
  ○ Type 1 (20% of RPGN): anti-GBM antibody disease.
  ○ Type 2 (25%): immune complex GN, which includes IgA nephropathy, postinfectious GN, lupus nephritis, and mixed cryoglobulinemia.
  ○ Type 3 (55%): pauci-immune (no immune deposits), which includes ANCA-associated vasculitis such as granulomatosis with polyangiitis (GPA; formerly Wegener granulomatosis), microscopic polyangiitis, and Churg-Strauss syndrome, as well as ANC-negative crescentic glomerulonephritis.
  ○ Type 4: Double Ab syndrome-features of both types 1 and 3.
- Patients present with renal insufficiency and glomerular hematuria, with variable amounts of proteinuria, edema, and hypertension.
- Serologic tests such as anti-GBM Ab, ANCA, ASO, ANA, hypocomplementemia, and cryocrit may point to a specific diagnosis.
- Renal biopsy is usually necessary for definitive diagnosis and to guide therapy.

## ■ Differential Diagnosis

- Anti-GBM antibody disease.
- ANCA-associated vasculitis.
- Lupus nephritis.
- IgA nephropathy.
- Mixed cryoglobulinemia.
- Membranoproliferative glomerulonephritis.

## ■ Treatment

- Though therapy is based on the specific disease implicated, most cases of RPGN are empirically treated with pulse steroids followed by oral steroids, and cyclophosphamide.
- Plasmapheresis is often used in patients with anti-GBM antibody disease, pulmonary hemorrhage, and in ANCA-associated vasculitis with severe renal disease.

## ■ Pearl

*When clinical suspicion for RPGN is high, intravenous steroid therapy should be initiated promptly; it will not affect the diagnostic utility of a renal biopsy.*

Reference

Little MA, Pusey CD: Rapidly progressive glomerulonephritis: current and evolving treatment Pauci-immune glomerulonephritis. J Nephrol 2004;17 Suppl 8:S10–19.

## Pulmonary Renal Syndrome

- **Essentials of Diagnosis**
  - Occurrence of pulmonary hemorrhage and acute renal failure due to an acute glomerulonephritis (typically a rapidly progressive glomerulonephritis).
  - Pulmonary hemorrhage is due to pulmonary capillaritis.
  - Pulmonary hemorrhage may be insidious and patients may present with iron deficiency anemia.
  - Pulmonary function tests show increased diffusion capacity for carbon monoxide (DLCO).
  - More than 50% of cases are ANCA positive.
  - Others are due to anti-GBM abs that deposit on glomerular and alveolar basement membranes (Goodpasture syndrome) and can be detected by linear staining of the GBM for IgG on renal biopsy.

- **Differential Diagnosis**
  - ANCA-associated vasculitis: granulomatosis with polyangiitis (GPA; formerly Wegener granulomatosis); microscopic polyangiitis; Churg-Strauss syndrome.
  - Anti-GBM disease (Goodpasture disease).
  - Systemic lupus erythematosis; cryoglobulinemic vasculitis; Henoch-Schonlein purpura.
  - Thrombotic microangiopathy.
  - Infective endocarditis with septic pulmonary emboli and immune complex glomerulonephritis.
  - Pulmonary edema with blood-tinged sputum with acute kidney injury.
  - Severe pneumonia with acute kidney injury.
  - Pulmonary embolism from venous thrombosis in patients with GPA.

- **Treatment**
  - Pulse steroids and plasma exchange initially, followed by oral prednisone and cyclophosphamide for Goodpasture disease and pauci-immmune glomerulonephritis.

- **Pearl**
*Prompt diagnosis and treatment is critical as pulmonary hemorrhage in anti-GBM and ANCA-associated disease may be life threatening.*

References

Merkel PA et al: Brief communication: high incidence of venous thrombotic events among patients with Wegener granulomatosis: The Wegener's Clinical Occurrence of Thrombosis (WeCLOT) study. Ann Intern Med 2005;142:620.

Niles JL et al: The syndrome of lung hemorrhage and nephritis is usually an ANCA-associated condition. Arch Intern Med 1996;156:440.

# Crescentic Glomerulonephritis

## ■ Essentials of Diagnosis
- The pathological hallmark of rapidly progressive glomerulonephritis–see chapter on RPGN.
- Classified according to immunofluorescence into three categories.
- Linear deposits of IgG on the glomerular basement membrane–anti-GBM disease.
- Few or no immune deposits (pauci-immune)–ANCA-associated disease.
- Granular deposits of immunoglobulin–immune complex disease.

## ■ Differential Diagnosis
- Linear deposits: Goodpasture disease or renal limited anti-GBM disease.
- Pauci-immune: granulomatosis with polyangiitis (GPA; formerly Wegener granulomatosis) microscopic polyangiitis (MPA), renal limited MPA.
- Immune complex: lupus nephritis, post-infectious GN, mixed cryoglobulinemia, Henoch-Schonlein nephritis, IgA nephropathy, membranoproliferative GN.

## ■ Treatment
- Varies according to the cause.
- Most causes are treated initially with pulse methylprednisolone.
- May include plasma exchange, cyclophosphamide, oral corticosteroids, rituximab for induction of remission and azathioprine, or mycophenolate mofetil for maintenance.
- Post-infectious causes are treated with appropriate antibiotics or antiviral agents.

## ■ Pearl
*Renal biopsy and immunofluorescence microscopy enable rapid diagnosis and treatment; serological tests provide further refinement.*

Reference

Little MA, Pusey CD: Rapidly progressive glomerulonephritis: current and evolving treatment strategies. J Nephrol 2004;17 Suppl 8:S10.

## Anti-glomerular Basement Membrane Disease

- **Essentials of Diagnosis**
  - Syndrome of rapidly progressive glomerulonephritis due to anti-glomerular basement membrane antibodies is called Goodpasture disease when it is accompanied by pulmonary hemorrhage.
  - Autoantibodies are directed against the noncollagenous domain (NC1) of the alpha 3 chain of type IV collagen (highly expressed in both the glomerular basement membrane and alveoli).
  - Bimodal age distribution with one peak at 20–30 years and second 50–70 years. Younger patients are more likely to be male and develop pulmonary and renal symptoms; older patients have equal sex distribution and have isolated glomerulonephritis.
  - Acute kidney injury with subnephrotic proteinuria and urinalysis showing dysmorphic RBCs or RBC casts, and WBCs.
  - Alveolar hemorrhage manifests as hemoptysis, dyspnea, and cough and is usually seen in smokers.
  - Light microscopy shows crescentic glomerulonephritis in most cases.
  - Immunofluorescence shows the classic linear deposition of IgG along the glomerular capillary walls.
  - 10–30% of patients will also test positive for ANCA.

- **Differential Diagnosis**
  - Granulomatosis with polyangiitis.
  - Microscopic polyangiitis.
  - Systemic lupus erythematosus.
  - Post-streptococcol glomerulonephritis.
  - Infective endocarditis.

- **Treatment**
  - Plasmapheresis to remove circulating anti-GBM antibodies combined with steroids and cyclophosphamide.
  - Patients requiring immediate dialysis or showing extensive crescents on biopsy are unlikely to have renal recovery despite treatment.
  - Plasmapheresis is indicated for patients with pulmonary hemorrhage regardless of renal function.
  - Untreated disease progresses to ESRD over weeks to months.
  - Generally low rate of recurrence in transplant patients if transplantation is delayed until anti-GBM antibody levels have been undetectable for 12 months.

- **Pearl**

*Iron deficiency and an elevated DLCO are clues to pulmonary hemorrhage.*

Reference

Pusey CD: Anti-glomerular basement membrane disease. Kidney Int 2003;64:1535.

## Goodpasture Syndrome

- **Essentials of Diagnosis**
  - A term originally used to denote the combination of acute glomerulonephritis and pulmonary alveolar hemorrhage; now reserved for those cases of anti-glomerular basement membrane (anti-GBM) nephritis accompanied by pulmonary hemorrhage.
  - Patients that have anti-GBM nephritis without pulmonary hemorrhage also fall under the diagnosis of Goodpasture disease.
  - Pulmonary symptoms include hemoptysis, dyspnea, fatigue, cough, fever, and chills.
  - Rapidly progressive glomerulonephritis (RPGN) is common.
  - C × R typically shows patchy or diffuse alveolar shadowing in the central lung fields and bronchoscopy may reveal hemorrhage.
  - DLCO is elevated due to hemoglobin in the alveolar spaces.
  - Light microscopy shows crescentic glomerulonephritis.
  - Immunofluorescence shows linear IgG deposits along the GBM.
  - Serologic evaluation should include anti-GBM titers and MPO and PR3 ANCA titers, streptozyme test, ANA, C3, and C4, and cryocrit to rule out other causes of RPGN.
  - Anti-GBM antibodies are reactive with the noncollagenous domain (NC1) of the alpha 3 chain of type IV collagen (expressed in the glomerular basement membrane and alveoli).

- **Differential Diagnosis**
  - Granulomatosis with polyangiitis.
  - Microscopic polyangiitis.
  - Systemic lupus erythematosus.
  - Churg-Strauss allergic granulomatosis.

- **Treatment**
  - Plasmapheresis to remove circulating anti-GBM antibodies, steroids, and cyclophosphamide should be initiated immediately.
  - Renal recovery may occur if treatment is initiated promptly. Patients requiring dialysis are unlikely to recover renal function despite treatment.
  - Plasmapheresis is indicated for patients with pulmonary hemorrhage regardless of renal function.
  - Untreated disease progresses to ESRD over weeks to months.
  - Generally low rate of recurrence if renal transplantation is delayed until anti-GBM antibody levels have been undetectable for 12 months.

- **Pearl**

*Treatment with plasmapheresis and immunosuppression is life saving in patients with pulmonary hemorrhage.*

Reference

Pusey C: Anti-glomerular basement membrane (anti-GBM) disease. Kidney Int 2003;64:1535.

## Renal Vasculitis

### ■ Essentials of Diagnosis
- Renal involvement common in systemic vasculitis.
- Wide range of clinical manifestations depending on vessels involved and organs affected.
- Large vessel vasculitis, mostly due to Takayasu arteritis, typically affect the aorta and renal arteries and cause renovascular hypertension.
- Medium vessel vasculitis, most commonly classic polyarteritis nodosa (PAN) involves medium-sized vessels and leads to renal failure, hypertension, renal infarction, and hemorrhage.
- Small vessel vasculitis involves the glomerular capillaries causing glomerulonephritis.
- An active urine sediment with dysmorphic red cells and red cell casts is seen in small vessel vasculitis, but not in medium and large vessel vasculitis.
- Renal biopsy in small vessel vasculitis shows a focal, necrotizing glomerulonephritis that is often crescentic.
- Angiography shows arterial stenosis in Takayasu arteritis and small intrarenal aneurysms in PAN.

### ■ Differential Diagnosis
- Large vessel vasculitis: Takayasu arteritis; giant cell arteritis.
- Medium vessel vasculitis: polyarteritis nodosa; Kawasaki disease in children.
- Small vessel vasculitis: Henoch-Schonlein purpura (IgA); cryo-globulinemic vasculitis; granulomatosis with polyangiitis (GPA; formerly Wegener granulomatosis); microscopic polyangiitis, and Churg-Straus Syndrome.

### ■ Treatment
- Immunosuppressive therapy usually with high-dose cortico-steroids initially, followed by a lower maintenance dose.
- Cryoglobulinemic vasculitis due to Hepatitis C infection and Hepatitis B–associated PAN may respond to antiviral treatment.

### ■ Pearl
*Always think of systemic vasculitis in a patient with AKI and multisystem disease with constitutional symptoms such as fever, weight loss, arthralgias, and myalgias.*

References

Hunder GG et al: The American College of Rheumatology 1990 criteria for the classification of vasculitis. Arthritis Rheum 1990;33:1065.

Samarkos M et al: The clinical spectrum of primary renal vasculitis. Semin Arthritis Rheum 2005;35:95.

## Pauci-immune Glomerulonephritis

- **Essentials of Diagnosis**
  - Necrotizing glomerulonephritis with little or no glomerular immunoglobulin deposits on immunofluorescence or electron microscopy.
  - Very common cause of rapidly progressive glomerulonephritis.
  - Renal failure at presentation.
  - May be anuric.
  - Variable degree of proteinuria.
  - Active sediment on urinalysis with hematuria, dysmorphic red cells, and red blood cell casts.
  - Typically due to a systemic small vessel vasculitis: granulomatosis with polyangiitis (GPA; formerly Wegener granulomatosis), microscopic polyangiitis, or Churg-Straus syndrome.
  - Most are ANCA-positive: 80% MPO-ANCA in renal-limited disease.
  - ANCA-negative patients have fewer extrarenal symptoms than those who are ANCA-positive.
  - Autoantibodies to lysosomal membrane protein-2 (LAMP-2) are a recently described ANCA subtype and are present in almost all individuals with pauci-immune glomerulonephritis.

- **Differential Diagnosis**
  - Granulomatosis with polyangiitis.
  - Microscopic polyangiitis.
  - Churg-Strauss syndrome.
  - "Renal-limited" vasculitis.
  - Drug-induced vasculitis; hydralazine; propylthiouracil; methimazole; penicillamine; allopurinol.
  - ANCA-negative pauci-immune glomerulonephritis.
  - Other causes of RPGN: Goodpasture syndrome/anti-glomerular basement membrane disease; immune complex GN.

- **Treatment**
  - Usually require pulse methylprednisolone at presentation.
  - Cyclophosphamide or Rituximab combined with corticosteroids.
  - Consider plasma exchange if severe disease requiring dialysis or if there is concurrent pulmonary hemorrhage.
  - Azathioprine or mycophenolate mofetil for maintenance therapy.

- **Pearl**

*Pauci-immune glomerulonephritis is the most common diagnosis in elderly patients presenting with acute kidney injury who undergo a renal biopsy.*

Reference

Chen M et al: ANCA-negative pauci-immune crescentic glomerulonephritis. Nat Rev Nephrol 2009;5:313.

## ANCA-Positive Renal Vasculitis

- **Essentials of Diagnosis**
  - Small vessel vasculitis syndromes associated with circulating antineutrophil cytoplasmic autoantibodies (ANCA), especially Granulomatosis with polyangiitis (GPA; formerly Wegener granulomatosis), systemic and renal-limited microscopic polyangiitis (MPA), and sometimes Churg-Strauss syndrome.
  - Clinical features include acute glomerulonephritis with renal failure and hematuria, arthralgias, skin rash, upper respiratory symptoms, and pulmonary hemorrhage.
  - Two types of ANCA assays: a sensitive indirect immunofluorescence (IF) assay and a more specific ELISA.
  - Testing is not standardized so there is considerable variability between laboratories.
  - Two patterns on IF: C-ANCA pattern (cytoplasmic staining) and P-ANCA (perinuclear staining).
  - ELISA directed against specific antigens: proteinase 3 (anti-PR3 = cANCA) and myeloperoxidase (anti-MPO = pANCA).
  - 80–90% of patients with GPA are ANCA positive – typically PR3-ANCA.
  - 70% of patients with MPA are ANCA positive – typically MPO-ANCA.
  - Anti-PR3 and anti-MPO have been detected with variable frequencies in Churg-Strauss syndrome.
  - Pathology shows focal necrotizing lesions involving arterioles, venules, and capillaries. Granulomas are seen in GPA.
  - Renal biopsy shows a pauci-immune necrotizing glomerulonephritis.

- **Differential Diagnosis**
  - Granulomatosis with polyangiitis.
  - Systemic microscopic polyangiitis.
  - Churg-Strauss syndrome.
  - "Renal-limited" vasculitis.
  - Drug-induced vasculitis: hydralazine, propylthiouracil, methimazole, penicillamine, allopurinol.
  - Other causes of rapidly progressive glomerulonephritis.

- **Treatment**
  - Cyclophosphamide or rituximab and glucocorticoids for induction therapy.
  - Plasma exchange in patients with severe renal disease; pulmonary hemorrhage and concurrent anti-GBM disease.
  - Maintenance therapy with azathioprine after 6 months of induction therapy with cyclophosphamide to prevent relapse.

- **Pearl**

*ANCA positivity occurs in 10–40% of patients with anti-GBM disease and is usually MPO-ANCA.*

References

Chen M, Kallenberg CG. ANCA-associated vasculitides–advances in pathogenesis and treatment. Nat Rev Rheumatol 2010;6:653–664.

# Granulomatosis with Polyangiitis
# (Formerly Wegener Granulomatosis)

## ■ Essentials of Diagnosis

- Systemic vasculitis associated with antineutrophil cytoplasmic antibodies (ANCA).
- Presents with acute or subacute renal failure associated with upper and/or lower respiratory tract symptoms.
- Microscopic hematuria with dysmorphic red cells and red cell casts on sediment.
- Subnephrotic to nephrotic range proteinuria.
- Although can have renal limited disease, most patients have respiratory symptoms including oral and/or nasal ulcers, recurrent sinusitis, dyspnea, cough, and hemoptysis with pulmonary nodules.
- May have conductive and sensorineural hearing loss.
- ANCA positive - typically anti-PR3 (c-ANCA); sometimes anti-MPO (p-ANCA).
- Biopsy at site of active disease reveals a necrotizing vasculitis with granulomatous inflammation.
- Renal biopsy shows focal necrotizing, pauci-immune glomerulonephritis with crescents in almost all cases.

## ■ Differential Diagnosis

- Microscopic polyangiitis.
- Churg-Strauss syndrome.
- Goodpasture syndrome/ anti-GBM disease.
- Henoch-Schonlein purpura.
- Cryoglobulinemic vasculitis.
- Systemic lupus erythematosus.
- Drug-induced vasculitis; hydralazine; propylthiouracil; methimazole; penicillamine; allopurinol.
- ANCA-negative pauci-immune glomerulonephritis

## ■ Treatment

- Cyclophosphamide or rituximab and glucocorticoids for induction therapy.
- Plasma exchange in patients with severe renal disease; pulmonary hemorrhage and concurrent anti-GBM disease.
- Maintenance therapy with azathioprine or mycophenolate mofetil.

## ■ Pearl

*Always examine the nasal septum in a patient with renal failure–a perforated septum should lead to consideration of cocaine use or granulomatosis with polyangiitis (formerly Wegener granulomatosis).*

### References

Jayne D et al: A randomized trial of maintenance therapy for vasculitis associated with antineutrophil cytoplasmic autoantibodies. N Engl J Med 2003;349:36.

Jayne DR et al: Randomized trial of plasma exchange or high-dosage methylprednisolone as adjunctive therapy for severe renal vasculitis. J Am Soc Nephrol 2007;18:2180.

Stone JH et al: Rituximab versus cyclophosphamide for ANCA-associated vasculitis. N Engl J Med 2010;363: 221.

# Microscopic Polyangiitis

- **Essentials of Diagnosis**
  - Systemic or renal limited vasculitis associated with anti-neutrophil cytoplasmic antibodies (ANCA).
  - Same spectrum of disease as granulomatosis with polyangiitis (GPA; formerly Wegener granulomatosis) except no granulomas are seen on biopsy.
  - Present with acute or subacute renal failure.
  - Microscopic hematuria with dysmorphic red cells and red cell casts on sediment.
  - Subnephrotic to nephrotic range proteinuria.
  - Differs from GPA in that the lungs are affected by a capillaritis rather than granulomata and upper respiratory involvement is less common.
  - ANCA positive - typically associated with MPO-ANCA.
  - Renal biopsy shows focal necrotizing pauci-immune glomerulonephritis with crescents in almost all cases.

- **Differential Diagnosis**
  - Granulomatosis with polyangiitis.
  - Churg-Strauss syndrome.
  - Goodpasture syndrome/ anti-GBM disease.
  - Henoch-Schonlein purpura (IgA).
  - Cryoglobulinemic vasculitis.
  - Systemic lupus erythematosus with nephritis.
  - Drug-induced vasculitis; hydralazine; propylthiouracil; methimazole; penicillamine; allopurinol.
  - ANCA-negative pauci-immune glomerulonephritis.

- **Treatment**
  - Cyclophosphamide or rituximab and glucocorticoids for induction therapy.
  - Plasma exchange in patients with severe renal disease, pulmonary hemorrhage, and/or concurrent anti-GBM disease.
  - Maintenance therapy with azathioprine or mycophenolate mofetil.

- **Pearl**

*Renal transplantation is effective for those patients with end-stage renal failure with a low recurrence rate.*

Reference

Pallan L et al: ANCA-associated vasculitis: from bench research to novel treatments. Nat Rev Nephrol 2009;278.

# Polyarteritis Nodosa

- ■ Essentials of Diagnosis
  - Necrotizing inflammation of medium or small arteries without glomerulonephritis or vasculitis of smaller vessels.
  - Rare disease with slight male predominance and age of onset between 40–60 years.
  - Most cases are idiopathic, but secondary PAN has been associated with Hepatitis B and C, and hairy cell leukemia.
  - ANCA is typically not present.
  - Renal involvement includes renal artery aneurysms, which can rupture; luminal narrowing of renal arteries leads to renal infarctions, activation of the renin-angiotensin system, and subsequent hypertension (30% of patients).
  - Renal insufficiency is common with subnephrotic proteinuria and minimal hematuria since the pathology is predominantly ischemic.
  - Renal symptoms can include flank pain and rarely, hematuria.
  - Arteriography may show small intrarenal arterial aneurysms and renal infarcts.
  - Renal biopsy shows segmental transmural fibrinoid necrosis of arteries with infiltrating leukocytes.
  - Diagnosis is based on clinical symptoms which affect numerous organs, angiographic findings, and tissue (not necessarily kidney) biopsy.

- ■ Differential Diagnosis
  - Malignant hypertension or scleroderma crisis.
  - Kawasaki disease.
  - Takayasu arteritis.

- ■ Treatment
  - Patients with only constitutional symptoms and normal renal function may be treated with steroids alone for 6–12 months.
  - More aggressive disease involving kidneys, heart, and CNS warrant cyclophosphamide in addition to steroids.
  - There is no role for plasmapheresis in idiopathic PAN.
  - Anti-viral therapy for hepatitis B when present together with immunosuppression and possibly plasmapheresis.

- ■ Pearl

*PAN causes renal ischemia, hypertension, and hemorrhage and should not be confused with microscopic polyangiitis which is a small vessel vasculitis that causes glomerulonephritis.*

Reference

Colmegna I et al: Polyarteritis nodosa revisited. Curr Rheumatol Rep 2005; 7(4):288.

## Hemolytic Uremic Syndrome

- **Essentials of Diagnosis**
  - Triad of microangiopathic hemolytic anemia, thrombocytopenia, and acute renal failure.
  - Most common in children under 5 years.
  - Two forms: D+HUS and D-HUS (atypical HUS) depending on association with preceding diarrheal illness.
  - D+HUS is usually due to infections with organisms producing a Shiga-like toxin: E. coli 0157:H7; Campylobacter, Shigella.
  - Circulating shiga toxin causes endothelial cell injury, thrombosis, and renal failure.
  - D-HUS (atypical HUS) may be familial or sporadic due to medications, infections (HIV), malignancy, transplantation, or pregnancy.
  - Abnormalities in the complement pathway underlie many cases of atypical HUS including complement factor H (CFH) mutations, deficiency, or antibodies against CFH.
  - Patients with atypical HUS may have low C3; normal C4.
  - Atypical HUS may be recurrent, frequently progresses to end-stage renal disease and is likely to recur after renal transplantation.
  - Drug induced: clopidogrel, ticlodipine, gemcitabine, mitomycin C, quinine, calcineurin inhibitors.
  - Renal biopsy shows fibrin platelet thrombi in the glomerular capillary lumina and arterioles and a membranoproliferative pattern of injury.

- **Differential Diagnosis**
  - TTP.
  - DIC.
  - Scleroderma renal crisis.
  - Catastrophic anti-phospholipid syndrome.
  - Pre-eclampsia/HELLP syndrome.
  - Malignant hypertension.

- **Treatment**
  - D+HUS in children is usually self-limited and requires only supportive therapy.
  - Stop possible causative drugs.
  - Plasma exchange for atypical HUS with CFH deficiency; corticosteroids and rituximab may help in those with antibodies against CFH; anti-C5 (eculizumab) for refractory cases.

- **Pearl**

*It is essential to distinguish between diarrhea-associated and atypical HUS as the prognosis and treatment differ.*

Reference

Noris M, Remuzzi G: Atypical hemolytic–uremic syndrome. N Engl J Med 2009;361:1676.

# Thrombotic Thrombocytopenic Purpura

■ **Essentials of Diagnosis**
- Classic pentad: fever; neurologic findings; microangiopathic hemolytic anemia; thrombocytopenia; and renal failure.
- Thrombocytopenia and microangiopathic hemolytic anemia occur in both TTP and HUS.
- Neurologic disease predominates in TTP; renal disease in HUS.
- Comprehensive term TTP-HUS increasingly being used.
- Microangiopathic hemolysis characterized by elevated LDH; low haptoglobin; and red cell fragmentation (schistocytes) on the peripheral blood smear.
- Renal disease often severe and may be anuric.
- Neurologic findings including headache, delirium, stroke, coma, and seizures.
- Deficiency of, or antibody against ADAMTS13, a von Willebrand factor cleaving protease causes ultra large vWF multimers to accumulate and cause platelet aggregation (platelet-rich clots) in affected organs.
- Not all the features of the pentad need be present in the same patient to diagnose TTP, and it should be considered in any patient with microangiopathic hemolytic anemia, thrombocytopenia, and renal failure.

■ **Differential Diagnosis**
- DIC, scleroderma renal crisis, pre-eclampsia/HELLP syndrome, catastrophic anti-phospholipid syndrome, malignant hypertension.

■ **Treatment**
- Plasma exchange: removes the antibody to ADAMTS13 and replaces ADAMTS13 with infusion of normal plasma.
- Platelet transfusion may exacerbate neurologic or renal complications.
- Immunosuppressive therapy with corticosteroids or rituximab for poorly responsive or relapsing disease.

■ **Pearl**

*Schistocytes may be seen on the peripheral smear of normal individuals and in renal disease, preeclampsia, and in patients with mechanical heart valves but only in TTP are more than 1% of RBCs schistocytes.*

Reference

Sadler JE: Von Willebrand factor, ADAMTS13, and thrombotic thrombocytopenic purpura. Blood 2008;112:11.

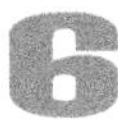

# Paraproteinemias

## Immunotactoid Glomerulopathy

### ■ Essentials of Diagnosis
- Evidence of renal disease (marked proteinuria and hematuria, impaired renal function).
- A renal biopsy showing glomerular deposits containing immunoglobulin by immunofluorescence that are Congo red negative and display a microtubular (20–35 nm in diameter) organized substructure by electron microscopy.
- Evidence by serum immunofixation, serum free light chains, immunofluorescence of glomerular deposits or bone marrow examinination indicating the presence of a neoplastic monoclonal plasma cell or lymphoproliferative disease.

### ■ Differential Diagnosis
- Immunotactoid glomerulopathy without a paraprotein disorder.
- Fibrillary glomerulonephritis.
- Cryoglobulinemic nephropathy.
- Membranoproliferative glomerulonephritis; Type I.
- Lupus Nephritis.

### ■ Treatment
- Uncertain. Chemotherapy (similar to that used for multiple myeloma or light chain deposition disease) may be helpful if a monoclonal paraproteinemia can be established. No randomized controlled trials available.
- High-dose (intravenous) methyl prednisolone and oral or IV cyclophosphamide in cases of rapidly progressive renal failure and extensive crescentic glomerulonephritis can be useful.
- Dialysis and renal transplantation (recurrent disease is a risk).

### ■ Pearl
*When a patient presents with apparently idiopathic nephrotic syndrome and a lesion of immunotactoid glomerulopathy is found on renal biopsy, an evaluation for monoclonal paraproteinemia should be undertaken.*

Reference

Schwartz MM et al: Immunotactoid glomerulopathy. J Am Soc Neprhol 2002;13:1390.

## Cast Nephropathy

- **Essentials of Diagnosis**
  - Evidence of multiple myeloma (lytic lesions on skeletal survey, anemia M-protein spike by immunofixation/immunoelectrophoresis of serum, abnormal number and neoplastic appearance of monoclonal plasma cells in the bone marrow and/or circulation).
  - Increased monoclonal light chains in urine.
  - Impaired renal function or acute renal failure.
  - Renal biopsy showing large glassy, fractured, weakly PAS positive casts in many tubules with tubular atrophy and focal interstitial inflammation (often giant cells around casts).

- **Differential Diagnosis**
  - Toxic acute kidney injury (anti-microbials, anti-neoplastic agents, bisphosphonates).
  - Hyperviscosity syndrome.
  - Hypercalcemia induced renal failure.
  - Collapsing glomerulopathy (bisphosphonate-induced).
  - Light chain deposition disease.
  - Extra-renal obstructive uropathy.
  - Hyperuricemic nephropathy (acute).

- **Treatment**
  - Chemotherapy for multiple myeloma (melphalan/dexamethasone; bortezomid/lenanilamide).
  - Dialysis, using high-flux membrane or peritoneal dialyses.
  - Intensive plasma exchange (controversial)—if light chains greatly elevated in circulation.
  - Loop diuretics and saline administration (caution if congestive heart failure present).

- **Pearl**

*Always consider cast nephropathy when acute kidney injury of uncertain origin presents in an older individual.*

### Reference

Cockwell P, Hutchinson CA: Management options for cast nephropathy in multiple myeloma. Curr Opin Nephrol Hypertens 2010;19:550.

# Light Chain Deposition Disease

## ■ Essentials of Diagnosis
- Clinical evidence of organ involvement (typically proteinuria with reduced renal function).
- Monoclonal light chains in serum and/or urine (typically kappa light chains by free light chain assay).
- Tissue (typically glomerular) deposits of monoclonal light chain. Congo red negative, amorphous or granular by electron microscopy, C3 negative.
- Absence of multiple myeloma by bone marrow examination, skeletal survey, or serum immunofixation.

## ■ Differential Diagnosis
- Multiple myeloma.
- Systemic amyloidosis.
- Heavy chain or light-heavy chain deposition diseases.
- Membranoproliferative glomerulonephritis; Types I and II (dense deposit disease).
- Fibrillary/immunotactoid glomerulopathy.
- Diabetic nodular glomerulosclerosis.
- Idiopathic nodular glomerulosclerosis.
- Chronic thrombotic microangiopathy.

## ■ Treatment
- Chemotherapy (chlorambucil or melphalan) plus steroids.
- Dialysis (for end-stage renal disease).
- Kidney transplantation (after control of the hematological disease).

## ■ Pearl
*Always consider light chain deposition disease in patients with heavy proteinuria and impaired renal function when a renal biopsy shows nodular intercapillary glomerulosclerosis.*

Reference

Lin J et al: Renal monoclonal immunoglobulin deposition disease: the disease spectrum. J Am Soc Nephrol 2001;12:1482.

## Primary Systemic Amyloidosis

- **Essentials of Diagnosis**
  - Clinical evidence of organ involvement (eg, proteinuria; reduced renal function, enlarged kidneys).
  - Monoclonal paraprotein in serum or urine (typically lambda light chain—by serum free light chain assay).
  - Tissue (eg, kidney, abdominal fat pad, rectal submucosal) deposits of AL amyloid (Congo red positive, lambda, or kappa light chain by immunofluorescence; 10–12 nonbranching fibrils by electron microscopy).
  - No evidence of plasma cell neoplasia (Multiple myeloma) by bone marrow biopsy, serum immunofixation or skeletal survey.

- **Differential Diagnosis**
  - Hereditary amyloidosis (fibrinogen alpha chain, lysozyme, lipoprotein A1, transthyretin—if deposits are Congo red positive, but negative for lambda or kappa light chains).
  - Secondary AA amyloidosis (rheumatoid arthritis; cancer; chronic infections; systemic auto-inflammatory disorders [eg, familial mediterranean fever] if deposits are Congo red positive, negative for lambda or kappa light chains and positive for AA Amyloid).
  - Multiple myeloma with AL amyloidosis.
  - Collapsing glomerulopathy (Congo red negative).
  - Immunotactoid/fibrillary glomerulonephritis (Congo red negative).
  - Advanced diabetic nephropathy (Congo red Negative).

- **Treatment**
  - High dose melphalan and dexamethasone.
  - Bortezomid and/or lenanilomide plus dexamethanose.
  - Modified chemotherapy and autologous stem cell transplantation (only for younger patients without multiple organ involvement, especially cardiac involvement).
  - Dialysis (for end-stage renal disease).
  - Kidney and/or heart transplantation.

- **Pearl**

*Always consider primary systemic amyloidosis in the differential diagnosis of apparently idiopathic nephrotic syndrome in a patient over the age of 50 years (especially with enlarged kidneys, easy bruising, carpal tunnel syndrome, cardiac disease, postural hypotension, or unexplained diarrhea)*

Reference

Sideras K, Gewtz MA: Amyloidosis. Adv Clin Chem 2009;47:1.

# 7

# Tubulointerstitial Diseases

## Acute Pyelonephritis

- ■ **Essentials of Diagnosis**
  - Presents with fever, chills, flank pain or costovertebral angle tenderness, and symptoms of cystitis.
  - Ascending infection from the urethra and bladder is the most common route of infection.
  - Risk factors for UTIs include female gender, frequent sexual intercourse, history of previous episodes of cystitis, pregnancy, diabetes, renal transplantation, older age, anatomical obstruction, vesicoureteral reflux, and urinary catheterization.
  - The most commonly identified urinary organisms are *Escherichia coli, Klebsiella pneumoniae, Enterococcus,* and *Proteus mirabilis.*
  - Urine Gram stain can help guide empiric antibiotic selection.
  - Pretreatment urine culture should be performed routinely in all patients with suspected pyelonephritis, with peripheral blood cultures in those requiring hospitalization.
  - Histopathologic findings are consistent with interstitial nephritis.

- ■ **Differential Diagnosis**
  - Similar presentations may occur in patients with renal calculus, gallbladder disease, hepatitis, pancreatitis, and appendicitis.

- ■ **Treatment**
  - If able to maintain oral intake, a 14-day course of oral fluoroquinolones is usually recommended (7 days if mild).
  - For more severe cases, intravenous fluoroquinolones, broad-spectrum cephalosporins (+/− aminoglycosides), carbapenems, or piperacillin-tazobactam may be used. Switch to oral medication can be made after clinical improvement.
  - Coverage of *Pseudomonas aeruginosa* should be considered.

- ■ **Pearl**

*The use of indwelling urinary catheters is an important modifiable risk factor for urinary tract infections and ultimately pyelonephritis.*

Reference

Ramakrishnan et al: Diagnosis and management of acute pyelonephritis in adults. Am Fam Physician 2005;72:2182.

## Acute Tubulointerstitial Nephritis

■ **Essentials of Diagnosis**
- Presents with acute kidney injury.
- Caused by medications (antibiotics, NSAIDs, PPIs), infections (pyelonephritis), and immune-mediated from systemic disorders.
- NSAID-related kidney injury can present as nephrotic syndrome with features of minimal change disease on renal biopsy or as membranous nephropathy. NSAIDs can also cause kidney injury through vasoconstriction of afferent arterioles in the kidney. NSAID-related kidney injury is more likely to be permanent than other causes.
- Fever, skin rash, and peripheral eosinophilia are seen in a minority of cases. Mild proteinuria, hematuria, sterile pyuria, and eosinophiluria may occur. Eosinophilia and eosinophiluria are not specific for acute tubulointerstitial nephritis.
- Findings associated with tubular dysfunction may be seen, including glycosuria, aminoaciduria, and wasting of potassium, magnesium, and salt. Renal tubular acidosis may be present.

■ **Differential Diagnosis**
- Acute tubulointerstitial nephritis is a clinical diagnosis. If clinically uncertain, renal ultrasound showing slight nephromegaly with increased echogenicity and gallium scan showing diffuse intense uptake bilaterally may be suggestive, limited by poor specificity.
- Renal biopsy (or if contraindicated, an empiric steroid trial) can help establish the diagnosis.

■ **Treatment**
- Discontinue the offending agent or treat the underlying infection.
- If no improvement in 10–15 days, pulsed methylprednisolone followed by oral prednisone tapered over 4–8 weeks is an accepted treatment. The optimal timing of steroids is unclear.
- Mycophenolate mofetil may be considered in steroid resistant or intolerant cases.

■ **Pearl**
*The diagnosis of acute tubulointerstitial nephritis requires a high index of suspicion. Consider it especially in patients using antibiotics or NSAIDs.*

Reference
Praga et al: Acute interstitial nephritis. Kidney Int 2010;77:956.

# Analgesic Nephropathy

## ■ Essentials of Diagnosis
- The most common cause of chronic interstitial nephritis.
- Associated with long-term ingestion of phenacetin, acetaminophen, aspirin, and caffeine. One gram of analgesics daily for 2 years is the minimum dose.
- Most common in women in their 60s or 70s.
- Symptoms and signs include chronic low back pain, chronic or recurrent headaches, chronic joint pains, and hypertension.
- Renal dysfunction is manifested by impaired urinary concentration, impaired sodium conservation, and renal tubular acidification defects.
- Urinalysis may show sterile pyuria, UTI, microscopic or macroscopic hematuria, and mild proteinuria.
- IV pyelogram reveals papillary necrosis, CT reveals papillary calcifications and "bumpy" renal contours, and ultrasound reveals small echogenic kidneys.
- Increased incidence of uroepithelial tumors and premature atherosclerosis.

## ■ Differential Diagnosis
- Other causes of chronic interstitial nephritis must be ruled out. A careful history of analgesic use combined with epidemiology may lend support to the diagnosis.

## ■ Treatment
- Management is supportive. The offending agent should be discontinued.
- New onset gross hematuria should raise suspicion for transitional cell cancer.

## ■ Pearl
*Analgesic nephropathy is the most common cause of chronic interstitial nephritis.*

### Reference
De Broe et al: Analgesic Nephropathy. N Engl J Med 1998;338:446.

## Balkan Nephropathy

- **Essentials of Diagnosis**
  - Balkan nephropathy is a form of chronic interstitial nephritis that slowly progresses to ESRD.
  - Familial.
  - Nearly all affected patients are farmers.
  - Normocytic, normochromic anemia is an early feature, more severe than expected for a given CKD stage. Later in disease, hypertension may develop.
  - Urinalysis shows mild proteinuria with few RBCs and WBCs.
  - Ultrasound may reveal bilaterally shrunken kidneys.
  - Patients are at increased risk of uroepithelial cancers.
  - Pathogenesis may be related to the flour obtained from wheat contaminated with seeds of the plant *Aristolochia clematis*.

- **Differential Diagnosis**
  - Diagnosis is based on epidemiology. Balkan nephropathy is endemic in the Balkan states, including former Yugoslavia, Bulgaria, and Romania.

- **Treatment**
  - Treatment is primarily supportive.

- **Pearl**

*Since treatment is primarily supportive, ensure that other causes of kidney injury have been ruled out before making this diagnosis in patients from the Balkan states.*

Reference

Stefanović et al: Fifty years of research in Balkan endemic nephropathy: Where are we now? Nephron Clin Pract 2009;112:c51.

## Chinese Herb Nephropathy

- **Essentials of Diagnosis**
  - Commonly seen among users of Chinese herbal medications for weight reduction.
  - Nephrotoxicity is usually attributed to aristolochic acid. Decline in renal function correlates with total dose received.
  - Affected patients usually have a normal blood pressure.
  - Pathology shows hypocellular interstitial fibrosis with marked tubular atrophy.
  - Increased incidence of uroepithelial tumors.

- **Differential Diagnosis**
  - Other causes of chronic interstitial nephritis may present similarly. Ascertaining the use of Chinese herbal medications containing aristolochic acid is the key to making the diagnosis.

- **Treatment**
  - A short course of oral steroids has been shown to slow progression of renal failure. If untreated, patients usually progress rapidly to end stage renal disease.

- **Pearl**

*Aristolochic acid nephropathy has been described in mostly middle-aged women in Belgium who were using Chinese herb pills as part of a weight loss regimen in 1992.*

Reference

Debelle et al: Aristolochic acid nephropathy: A worldwide problem. Kidney Int 2008;74:158.

## Chronic Pyelonephritis

- **Essentials of Diagnosis**
  - Chronic pyelonephritis is the term given to chronic infection-associated kidney injury not caused by vesicoureteral reflux (VUR), which is termed reflux nephropathy.
  - Chronic urinary tract infections are a common cause of chronic interstitial nephritis.
  - Patients typically present with fever, chills, dysuria, flank or back pain, and hypertension.
  - Distal tubular dysfunction may occur, characterized by acidosis and hyperkalemia.
  - Histopathologically, findings are similar to other forms of CIN.

- **Differential Diagnosis**
  - The presence of vesicoureteral reflux must be evaluated and other causes of chronic interstitial nephritis should be ruled out prior to making a diagnosis of chronic pyelonephritis.
  - Xanthogranulomatous pyelonephritis is a localized infection that can develop when chronic pyelonephritis persists. Underlying urinary tract obstruction (eg, nephrolithiasis) may become complicated by infection, renal ischemia, accumulation of lipid-laden macrophages (termed foam cells), and subsequent granuloma formation.

- **Treatment**
  - Urinary tract infection, if present, should be adequately treated.

- **Pearl**

*In any patient with suspected chronic pyelonephritis, consider imaging to evaluate for vesicoureteral reflux and xanthogranulomatous pyelonephritis, as nephrectomy may be necessary in these cases.*

Reference

Kuo et al: Xanthogranulomatous pyelonephritis: Critical analysis of 30 patients. Int Urol Nephrol 2010 Jun 11. [Epub ahead of print]

# Chronic Tubulointerstitial Nephritis

## ■ Essentials of Diagnosis
- Chronic tubulointerstitial nephritis is the name given to acute tubulointerstitial nephritis that has failed to resolve or has been resistant to treatment. It can also arise from chronic or intermittent low-grade injury to the tubulointerstitium.
- Functional abnormalities depend on the area of the tubule that is involved, with distal tubule dysfunction characterized by acidosis and hyperkalemia, and renal medullary dysfunction characterized by an inability to concentrate urine.
- Concomitant glomerular abnormalities may develop as chronic tubulointerstitial nephritis progresses.
- Histopathologically, interstitial chronic inflammation, interstitial fibrosis, and/or tubular atrophy may be seen.

## ■ Differential Diagnosis
- CIN may be caused by primary (idiopathic) or secondary etiologies.
- Primary causes include Epstein-Barr virus.
- Secondary causes include infections (BK virus, pyelonephritis), medications (analgesics, lithium, acyclic nucleoside inhibitors, calcineurin inhibitors, aristolochic acid, chemotherapeutic agents, acute phosphate nephropathy), heavy metals (cadmium, lead), hematologic diseases (multiple myeloma, lymphoproliferative disorders, light chain disease, sickle cell nephropathy), obstructive and reflux nephropathy, immune-mediated (sarcoid, Sjögren, TINU syndrome, idiopathic hypocomplementemic interstitial nephritis), metabolic (hyperoxaluria, hypercalcemia, hypercalciuria, chronic hypokalemia), genetic (cystinosis, Dent disease), and miscellaneous (Balkan nephropathy, radiation nephritis).

## ■ Treatment
- Treatment depends on the underlying etiology.

## ■ Pearl
*The differential diagnosis for chronic tubulointerstitial nephritis is very broad. A thorough workup is necessary to establish an underlying diagnosis and to guide treatment.*

Reference

Tanaka et al: Pathogenesis of tubular interstitial nephritis. Contrib Nephrol 2011;169:297.

# Cystinuria

- **Essentials of Diagnosis**
  - Autosomal, recessive disorder associated with defective transport of cystine, ornithine, lysine, and arginine in the renal tubule epithelium and GI tract. Types A and B cystinuria affect different genes, with Type A being more severe.
  - Presents with cystine ureteral stones, which may lead to urinary tract infections and renal failure.
  - Males more severely affected than females, though prevalence is equal among genders.
  - Definitive diagnosis requires demonstration of hexagonal cystine crystals in the urine. Acidification of concentrated urine with acetic acid can precipitate crystals not visible on initial urine microscopy.
  - The cyanide nitroprusside test may be performed on urine, resulting in a red/purple color if cystine is present in the urine.
  - Cystine stones appear radiopaque on imaging.

- **Differential Diagnosis**
  - Patients with magnesium ammonium phosphate and calcium stones may also present concurrently with urinary tract infections, leading to a similar clinical picture.

- **Treatment**
  - Increasing fluid intake (up to 4 L/d) and reducing sodium in the diet may result in lower urinary cystine concentrations.
  - Urinary alkalinization with potassium citrate may increase the solubility of cystine and decrease the risk of nephrolithiasis.
  - D-penicillamine can bind to the cysteine molecules making up cystine to form a penicillamine-cystine complex that is much more soluble than cystine. Mercaptopropionylglycine works similarly.
  - Kidney transplantation may be necessary if progression to ESRD occurs. A kidney from an unaffected donor will not form cystine stones.
  - Extracorporeal shock wave lithotripsy is not helpful.

- **Pearl**

*"Cys" sounds like "six." Cystine stones are hexagonal.*

**Reference**
Mattoo et al: Cystinuria. Semin Nephrol 2008;28:181.

## Dent Disease

- **Essentials of Diagnosis**
  - An x-linked recessive disease caused by mutations in the *CLCN5* gene.
  - Renal failure is seen only in males. Females have an attenuated phenotype.
  - Clinical manifestations include hypercalciuria with calcium phosphate nephrolithiasis, rickets, osteomalacia, nephrocalcinosis, low-molecular-weight proteinuria, and renal failure.
  - A primary Fanconi syndrome, manifesting with hypokalemia, aminoaciduria, and glycosuria may be evident.
  - Renal biopsy reveals a pattern of chronic interstitial nephritis with scattered calcium deposits.

- **Differential Diagnosis**
  - The X-linked recessive pattern of inheritance can help distinguish Dent disease from other processes causing chronic interstitial nephritis. Of note, the same mutation can induce different phenotypes in different families.

- **Treatment**
  - Renal stones and hypercalciuria are managed by increasing fluid intake.
  - Thiazide diuretics may be given in small doses but may cause hypotension and excessive diuresis.
  - Vitamin D supplementation may be used cautiously to treat rickets and osteomalacia, but it may worsen hypercalciuria.
  - Dietary calcium restriction is not recommended as it may exacerbate bone disease.

- **Pearl**

*Renal failure affecting only men is no accident.*

Reference

Devuyst et al: Dent's disease. Orphanet J Rare Dis 2010;5:28.

## Granulomatous Interstitial Nephritis (GIN)

- **Essentials of Diagnosis**
  - GIN is a rare histologic diagnosis that is present in 0.5–0.9% of native renal biopsies and 0.6% of renal transplant biopsies.
  - Patients may present with advanced renal failure and minimal proteinuria.
  - GIN has been associated with medication, infections, sarcoidosis, crystal deposits, paraproteinemias, and granulomatosis with polyangiitis (formerly Wegener granulomatosis). It has been described in a cause of TINU syndrome but can also be idiopathic.
  - Possible medications causing GIN include anticonvulsants, antibiotics, NSAIDs, allopurinol, and diuretics.
  - Mycobacteria and fungi are common infective causes and represent the main causative factors in renal transplants with GIN.

- **Differential Diagnosis**
  - GIN is a histologic diagnosis that requires a work-up for the underlying cause, with potential etiologies outlined above.

- **Treatment**
  - Once infective causes have been ruled out, corticosteroids represent the first-line treatment.
  - Steroid-sparing agents may be considered in cases where relapse occurs after withdrawal of steroids.

- **Pearl**

*Make sure to rule out tuberculosis in any patient with suspected GIN before initiating steroids.*

### Reference

Joss et al: Granulomatous interstitial nephritis. Clin J Am Soc Nephrol 2007;2:222.

# Lead Nephropathy

## ■ Essentials of Diagnosis

- Lead accumulates in proximal tubules, causing Fanconi syndrome and a decrease in GFR.
- Lead nephropathy is frequently associated with gout.
- The diagnosis is established via the EDTA mobilization test. Two grams of EDTA is administered IV/IM, with subsequent measurement of 24-hour urine lead excretion. Urinary lead more than 0.6 g/d is considered abnormal. One major limitation of this test is that it cannot mobilize lead deposits in bone. X-ray fluorescence can be used to determine bone lead content.
- Reduced levels of erythrocyte aminolevulinate dehydrase (ALAD) compared to levels of ALAD "restored" by the addition of dithiothreitol may be even more efficient in detecting increased body lead burden in patients with chronic kidney disease.
- With years of lead exposure, histopathology reveals progressive tubular atrophy and widespread fibrosis. Renal biopsy may reveal nonspecific findings seen in chronic interstitial nephritis.

## ■ Differential Diagnosis

- Other causes of chronic interstitial nephritis must be ruled out. Other symptoms of lead toxicity, including anemia, peripheral neuropathy, encephalopathy, and gout may suggest the diagnosis of lead nephropathy in a patient with kidney injury.

## ■ Treatment

- EDTA chelation therapy or oral succimer have been shown to slow the progression of chronic kidney disease.

## ■ Pearl

*Serum levels of lead may be elevated during acute exposure but are not very helpful in the chronically exposed.*

### Reference

Ekong et al: Lead-related nephrotoxicity: A review of the epidemiologic evidence. Kidney Int 2006;70:2074.

## Lithium Toxicity

- **Essentials of Diagnosis**
  - Chronic interstitial nephritis is the most common pathologic finding in chronic lithium nephropathy.
  - Typically, renal dysfunction is mild to moderate. However, patients with serum creatinine levels more than 2.5 mg/dL on presentation often progress to ESRD.
  - Polydipsia and polyuria suggest the onset of nephrogenic diabetes insipidus.
  - Incomplete distal renal tubular acidosis (RTA) occurs in up to 50% of patients.
  - Lithium has also been associated with hypercalcemia, potentially through its activity in the parathyroid gland.
  - Pathology shows cystic dilation of the distal tubules, with formation of "microcysts".
  - Increased incidence of uroepithelial tumors.

- **Differential Diagnosis**
  - Other causes of chronic interstitial nephritis must be ruled out. Duration of treatment with lithium correlates with development of nephrogenic diabetes insipidus (average 6.5–10 years) and ESRD (average 20 years).

- **Treatment**
  - Dose reduction or complete withdrawal of lithium is the mainstay of therapy.
  - Amiloride has been shown to reduce polyuria and to block lithium uptake in the sodium channels of the collecting duct.
  - Though thiazides may reduce lithium-induced polyuria, they may cause intravascular volume depletion, which can aggravate acute lithium toxicity through increasing reabsorption of sodium (and thereby lithium as well).

- **Pearl**

*Polydipsia and polyuria are the first symptoms suggesting development of lithium-related kidney toxicity.*

Reference

Grünfeld et al: Lithium nephrotoxicity revisited. Nat Rev Nephrol 2009;5:270.

## Papillary Necrosis

### ■ Essentials of Diagnosis

- Renal papillary necrosis is the result of an ischemic process in the renal papillae. Renal papillary necrosis is a pathologic finding, not a diagnosis.
- May be caused by diabetes, analgesic abuse or overuse, sickle cell disease, pyelonephritis, renal vein thrombosis, tuberculosis, and obstructive uropathy.
- Headaches and upper gastrointestinal symptoms may present early. Later symptoms/signs include nocturia, dysuria, bacteriuria, pyuria, microscopic hematuria, ureteral colic, and lower back pain. Clinical pathology may reveal decreased GFR and RTA.
- Complications include hypertension, cardiac disease, peripheral vascular disease, renal calculi, and bladder stones.
- Findings consistent with renal papillary necrosis are best visualized on intravenous urography and contrast-enhanced CT imaging. Ultrasonography findings are suggestive but not specific.

### ■ Differential Diagnosis

- As renal papillary necrosis is not a diagnosis in itself, a thorough workup is needed to identify the underlying cause.

### ■ Treatment

- Treatment depends on the underlying etiology.

### ■ Pearl

*In England and Australia, renal papillary necrosis has been reported to account for 15–20% of patients needing renal transplants.*

References

Brix: Renal papillary necrosis. Toxicology Pathology 2002;30:672.

Jung et al: Renal papillary necrosis: Review and comparison of findings at multi-detector row CT and intravenous urography. Radiographics 2006;26:1827.

## Primary Hyperoxaluria

- **Essentials of Diagnosis**
  - Rare, autosomal recessive genetic disorder due to deficiency of an oxalate-metabolizing liver enzyme.
  - Patients present with gross hematuria and renal colic during childhood.
  - Excessive oxalate in the urinary tract combines with calcium to form calcium oxalate, resulting in nephrolithiasis and chronic interstitial nephritis.
  - Majority of patients progressing to end-stage renal disease by the second decade of life.
  - Polarized light microscopy demonstrates birefringent positive crystals in the interstitial spaces and tubular lumens with surrounding inflammation and interstitial fibrosis.

- **Differential Diagnosis**
  - Other causes of chronic interstitial nephritis must be considered.

- **Treatment**
  - Maintaining a high urine flow may be beneficial to prevent nephrolithiasis.
  - The recommended treatment for those with recurrent nephrolithiasis or end-stage renal disease is combined liver and kidney transplantation.
  - Pyridoxine has been used with some success.

- **Pearl**

*If renal transplant is performed without concurrent liver transplant, hyperoxaluria will persist, leading to recurrence of nephrolithiasis and renal failure.*

**Reference**

Hoppe et al: The primary hyperoxalurias. Kidney Int 2009;75:1264.

# Radiation Nephritis

- ## Essentials of Diagnosis
  - Symptoms include edema, hypertension, proteinuria (which may be marked in acute radiation nephritis), acute kidney injury, and microangiopathic hemolytic anemia.
  - Acute radiation nephritis usually presents 6–12 months after radiation exposure, whereas chronic radiation nephritis typically presents more than 18 months after radiation exposure.
  - Radiation may cause direct injury to the tubular epithelial cells, and at higher doses may cause endothelial cell injury resulting in chronic ischemic injury to the kidneys. Concomitant chemotherapy may potentiate radiation-induced kidney injury.
  - Histopathologically, characteristic findings include thickening of the capillary walls with "splitting," where there is interposition of deposits between split layers of the glomerular basement membrane similar to HUS and TTP.
  - Prevention consists of proper shielding of the kidneys, dividing the total irradiation dose into smaller doses over a longer duration, and minimizing the total irradiation dose when possible.

- ## Differential Diagnosis
  - For patients receiving concurrent chemotherapy, chemotherapy-induced kidney injury should be considered. Common drugs implicated are cisplatin, ifosfamide, and carmustine. Other causes of chronic interstitial nephritis may present in a similar fashion.

- ## Treatment
  - ACE inhibitors are the recommended agents in the setting of hypertension.

- ## Pearl

*In cancer patients with kidney injury, always consider chemotherapy-induced kidney toxicity and radiation nephritis.*

### Reference

Dawson et al: Radiation-associated kidney injury. Int J Radiat Oncol Biol Phys 2010;76(3 Suppl):S108.

## Reflux Nephropathy

- **Essentials of Diagnosis**
  - Can occur congenitally or can be acquired.
  - Congenital nephropathy associated with vesicoureteral reflux (VUR) occurs in the absence of infection. With routine prenatal ultrasonography, many children with VUR are detected prior to the development of a UTI. The incidence of VUR in patients with prenatally diagnosed hydronephrosis is 15–20%. More common in boys than girls.
  - Acquired reflux-associated nephropathy is defined by renal scarring associated with intrarenal reflux of infected urine. Among young children, there is a 4:1 female predominance, and in older children the incidence is equivalent between genders.
  - Intravenous urography (IVU) was used in the past to detect renal scars, but this has now been largely replaced by the technetium 99m dimercaptosuccinic acid (DMSA) nuclear scan. Whereas IVU only provides structural information, a DMSA scan is able to provide a functional assessment.
  - The major complications of reflux nephropathy are hypertension and renal impairment.

- **Differential Diagnosis**
  - Chronic pyelonephritis and xanthogranulomatous pyelonephritis may present in a similar fashion. Imaging can help distinguish these entities.

- **Treatment**
  - Aggressive treatment of hypertension, prevention of breakthrough UTIs, and the use of ACEIs can decrease the rate of renal deterioration and preserve renal function.
  - Nephrectomy can also be useful in the treatment of hypertension if the source of hypertension can be lateralized.

- **Pearl**

*In any patient with recurrent pyelonephritis, consider imaging to evaluate for vesicoureteral reflux and xanthogranulomatous pyelonephritis, as nephrectomy may be necessary in these cases.*

Reference

Peters et al: Vesicoureteral reflux associated renal damage: congenital reflux nephropathy and acquired renal scarring. J Urol 2010;184:265.

## Retroperitoneal Fibrosis

### ■ Essentials of Diagnosis

- Retroperitoneal fibrosis (RF) is a rare fibrosing disorder that usually affects periaortic and periiliac retroperitoneal soft tissues, often resulting in obstructive uropathy.
- RF has an insidious clinical onset characterized by flank, back or abdominal pain, and constitutional symptoms such as malaise, fever, anorexia, and weight loss.
- Laboratory findings often reveal high ESR and CRP levels; auto-antibodies are also sometimes positive.
- Ureteral obstruction causing acute or chronic renal insufficiency is the most common and severe complication of RF.
- About 80–100% of RF patients show ureteral involvement, usually bilateral.
- CT and MRI typically reveal a periaortic mass of soft-tissue density extending from the level of the renal arteries to the iliac vessels and frequently causing medial ureteral deviation and obstruction; atypical peripancreatic, periureteral, or pelvic localizations have also been reported.
- Histologic examination of the retroperitoneal tissue is still the most reliable diagnostic tool because it may rule out other lesions of malignant, benign, or infectious origin.

### ■ Differential Diagnosis

- Differential includes retroperitoneal lymphoma, sclerosing mesenteritis, desmoid-type fibromatosis, inflammatory myofibroblastic tumor, Erdheim–Chester disease, and well-differentiated liposarcoma, sclerosing variant.

### ■ Treatment

- Administration of steroids (and/or steroid-sparing agents) is the first line of treatment. Tamoxifen has been shown to be beneficial in small trials. Optimal length of therapy has not been well-defined.
- Ureteral stenting and percutaneous nephrostomy are temporizing measures if obstructive uropathy is present. This may be followed by ureterolysis, an open surgical procedure.

### ■ Pearl

*Adequate tissue sampling to rule out malignancy is necessary prior to initiating corticosteroids.*

Reference

Corradi et al: Idiopathic retroperitoneal fibrosis: Clinicopathologic features and differential diagnosis. Kidney Int 2007;72:742.

## Scleroderma

- **Essentials of Diagnosis**
  - Manifests either as a slowly progressive chronic renal disease or as scleroderma renal crisis (SRC).
  - SRC is characterized by acute kidney injury, malignant hypertension, and rapidly progressive oliguric renal failure. Microangiopathic hemolytic anemia, thrombocytopenia, and elevated plasma renin activity may occur during episodes of SRC.
  - Urinalysis reveals proteinuria, microscopic hematuria, and granular casts.
  - One-year survival rates are approximately 70% with appropriate treatment.

- **Differential Diagnosis**
  - Making a diagnosis of scleroderma is the key to subsequent diagnosis of scleroderma renal crisis. The cutaneous symptoms of systemic sclerosis typically predate renal injury. The presence of Raynaud phenomenon, telangiectasias, arthralgias, myopathy, esophageal dysmotility, pulmonary fibrosis, myocardial fibrosis, and pericarditis should raise suspicion for SRC in the setting of kidney injury.

- **Treatment**
  - ACE inhibitors are the mainstay of therapy. Additional antihypertensives may be needed. Blood pressure should be lowered gradually (10–20 mm Hg/d) to avoid renal hypoperfusion.
  - ARBs have not been found to be as helpful. Avoid diuretics.
  - Peritoneal and hemodialysis are options for ESRD.
  - Kidney transplantation may be offered, though graft survival rates may be worse than other causes of ESRD, and there is a risk of recurrence of SRC in the transplanted kidney.

- **Pearl**

*Ten percent of all scleroderma patients (and 25% of those with systemic sclerosis) develop SRC within 4 years of diagnosis of scleroderma.*

Reference

Penn et al: Diagnosis, management and prevention of scleroderma renal disease. Curr Opin Rheumatol 2008;20:692.

## Secondary Hyperoxaluria

- ■ **Essentials of Diagnosis**
  - Patients present with gross hematuria and renal colic.
  - May result from ingestion of sour "star fruit," chronic diarrhea (via decreased intestinal calcium availability and excessive reabsorption of unbound oxalate in the GI tract), and excessive ascorbic acid intake (via metabolization into glyoxylate and oxalate).
  - Chronic diarrhea-related hyperoxaluria is termed enteric hyperoxaluria and is commonly seen in patients who have undergone extensive small bowel resections or jejunoileal bypass procedures.
  - Excessive oxalate in the urinary tract combines with calcium to form calcium oxalate, resulting in nephrolithiasis and chronic interstitial nephritis.
  - Polarized light microscopy demonstrates birefringent positive crystals in the interstitial spaces and tubular lumens with surrounding inflammation and interstitial fibrosis.

- ■ **Differential Diagnosis**
  - Other causes of chronic interstitial nephritis must be considered.

- ■ **Treatment**
  - A low fat, low oxalate diet is recommended.
  - Oral calcium carbonate and cholestyramine both bind intestinal oxalate and may be of some use.
  - Ascorbic acid intake should be limited.

- ■ **Pearl**

*The reason why a low fat diet may be helpful is that luminal free fatty acids promote the permeability of colon epithelium to oxalate, increasing oxalate absorption.*

Reference

Hoppe et al: Diagnostic and therapeutic approaches in patients with secondary hyperoxaluria. Front Biosci 2003;8:e437.

## Sickle Cell Nephropathy

- **Essentials of Diagnosis**
  - Presents with microscopic and gross hematuria (>50%), renal papillary necrosis (15–36%), proteinuria (26–40%), progressive renal failure (5%), nephrotic syndrome (3%), and polyuria.
  - Sickling in the medullary microcirculation may cause impaired urinary concentration and distal RTA.
  - Onset typically occurs after age 30, with 50% progressing to ESRD within 2 years and death within 4 years despite dialysis.
  - Highly aggressive renal cell carcinoma has been described in some patients with sickle cell disease.

- **Differential Diagnosis**
  - Urinary tract infection, rhabdomyolysis, renal vein thrombosis, and intravascular hemolysis can all occur in patients with sickle cell disease and may present with renal injury.

- **Treatment**
  - Triggers of sickling (eg, infection, dehydration, hypoxia, and cold) should be avoided.
  - ACE inhibitors should be used to treat proteinuria to slow renal disease progression.
  - Dialysis is commonly used. Transplantation portends better patient survival than hemodialysis.
  - One-year survival rates after kidney transplantation are similar to other causes of ESRD but there is a trend toward lower allograft survival thereafter.

- **Pearl**

*Though hydroxyurea is helpful in the prevention of pain crisis, it is not known whether fewer sickle cell crises translates to a lower incidence of renal disease.*

Reference

Scheinman et al: Sickle cell disease and the kidney. Nat Clin Pract Nephrol 2009;5:78.

# Tubulointerstitial Nephritis with Uveitis (TINU) Syndrome

## ■ Essentials of Diagnosis
- Patients present with nonspecific signs and symptoms (ie, fever, malaise), acute kidney injury, and anterior uveitis bilaterally (eye pain and redness, blurry vision, photophobia).
- Renal manifestations include both proximal and distal tubular dysfunction.
- Uveitis can occur as quickly as 2 months prior to, simultaneously with, or up to 14 months after the onset of interstitial nephritis.
- Commonly affects young adult women and adolescents.
- Pathology shows a predominance of CD4 and CD8 T lymphocytes.
- Ultrasonography may reveal bilateral nephromegaly.
- Pathogenesis may involve a delayed type hypersensitivity reaction to *Chlamydia* and EBV in the setting of suppressed cell-mediated immunity.

## ■ Differential Diagnosis
- Other common causes of tubulointerstitial disease that may present with uveitis including sarcoidosis and Sjögren syndrome.

## ■ Treatment
- Renal disease frequently resolves spontaneously without steroids but may take up to a year.
- For those with chronic kidney disease, prednisone 40–60 mg/d can be given for 3–6 months and tapered subsequently. A prolonged course of treatment is needed in TINU as renal relapses are frequent.
- Uveitis may not respond readily to steroid therapy and may require more aggressive therapy. For uveitis alone, topical steroids are an option.

## ■ Pearl
*The presence of redness and pain over the eyes, blurry vision, or photophobia in any patient with acute kidney injury should raise suspicion for TINU syndrome.*

Reference

Parameswaran et al: Tubulointerstitial nephritis with uveitis syndrome: A case report and review of literature. Indian J Nephrol 2010;20:103.

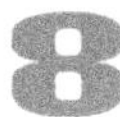

# Vascular Diseases of the Kidneys

# Atheroembolic Renal Disease

## ■ Essentials of Diagnosis

- Acute, subacute, or chronic kidney disease resulting from occlusion of renal vessels by cholesterol emboli from atherosclerotic plaques of the aorta or other major arteries.
- Atheroembolization can affect several organ systems, including the skin, gastrointestinal tract, and central nervous system. Skin lesions, such as livedo reticularis or cyanotic, cold and painful toes, are the most common extrarenal manifestation.
- Although spontaneous atheroembolism can occur, this disease is more frequently iatrogenic, developing after vascular procedures (most commonly angiography), anticoagulation or thrombolysis.
- Transient eosinophilia commonly occurs during the acute phase.
- Urinalysis usually reveals few cells and minimal protein uria.
- Renal biopsy is the definitive diagnostic method; biopsy of skin lesions is less invasive and has a high diagnostic yield.

## ■ Differential Diagnosis

- Small vessel vasculitis can be distinguished from renal atheroemboli by ANCA testing and by the urine sediment, which is usually bland with atheroemboli and nephritic in vasculitis.
- With contrast nephropathy after a radiologic procedure, the serum creatinine peaks within a few days and returns to baseline in 10–14 days, whereas atheroemboli usually causes progressive kidney injury over several weeks after the inciting event.
- Eosinophilia may be found in acute interstitial nephritis, but this condition also has an active urine sediment and should be suspected when acute kidney injury, fever, and skin rash follow treatment with an offending drug.

## ■ Treatment

- Avoidance of exposures that could cause further embolic events.
- Aggressive medical management of hypertension, cardiovascular disease, and renal failure (dialysis is necessary in some cases).
- Steroids may be beneficial, but their use is controversial.
- Statins may lower the risk of developing ESRD.

## ■ Pearl

*In patients with acute or subacute kidney injury following a precipitating event (eg, coronary angiography) and classic skin findings, a clinical diagnosis of atheroembolic renal disease can be made without a renal biopsy. Patients in whom fundoscopic exam reveals cholesterol crystals in the retinal vessels can also be diagnosed without tissue sampling.*

### Reference
Scolari F, Ravani P: Atheroembolic renal disease. Lancet 2010;375:1650.

## Renal Artery Aneurysm (RAA)

### ■ Essentials of Diagnosis
- Most patients are asymptomatic, and RAAs are usually diagnosed incidentally on imaging studies performed for other reasons.
- Some patients may have nonspecific flank or abdominal pain, hematuria, or an abdominal bruit.
- RAAs may initially present with a complication, the most serious of which is aneurysm rupture, which can lead to loss of ipsilateral renal function, hemorrhagic shock, and death.
- Other complications include renovascular hypertension, thrombosis causing arterial occlusion, and distal embolization.
- Radiographic diagnosis can be made with renal angiography or MRA; CT has been used for monitoring known aneurysms.

### ■ Differential Diagnosis
- Saccular aneurysms, the most common type, are usually extrarenal but may be located anywhere along the vascular tree.
- Fusiform aneurysms usually follow areas of stenosis, and are frequently associated with fibromuscular dysplasia.
- Intrarenal aneurysms, which are much less common than extrarenal aneurysms and frequently multiple, may be congenital, posttraumatic (eg, following renal biopsy) or associated with arteritis (eg, polyarteritis nodosa).

### ■ Treatment
- Data from specialized centers show high rates of long-term arterial patency after surgical correction, with improvement or complete resolution of hypertension in some patients.
- Expert recommendations for surgery include RAA diameter more than 1.5–2 cm in normotensive patients, or more than 1 cm in patients with difficult to control hypertension or in women who may become pregnant, concurrent renal artery stenosis, evidence of distal embolization, or expansion on follow-up imaging.
- Other patients may be monitored by CT or MRI every 1–2 years.

### ■ Pearl
*The risk of RAA rupture is increased during pregnancy, with most cases occurring during the last trimester. This diagnosis should be considered in pregnant women with acute onset of abdominal or flank pain, and nephrectomy may be required to control bleeding.*

References

Renal artery aneurysms. In: Schrier RW, ed. Diseases of the Kidney & Urinary Tract. 8th ed. Philadelphia: Lippincott Williams & Wilkins; 2007:1793.

Henke PK et al: Renal artery aneurysms. Ann Surg 2001;234:454.

# Renal Artery Dissection

## ■ Essentials of Diagnosis

- Acute dissections commonly present with abdominal or flank pain, as well as with new or worsening hypertension. Some patients have nausea and vomiting.
- Hematuria and worsening renal function may be present depending on the degree of renal ischemia caused by the dissection.
- The cases of most severe ischemia may result in renal infarction with irreversible loss of renal function.
- Chronic dissections most frequently present with renovascular hypertension but are usually otherwise asymptomatic.
- The diagnosis may be made by MRA or renal angiography.

## ■ Differential Diagnosis

- Acute dissections are generally of 2 types: spontaneous dissections, which are often associated with atherosclerosis; and iatrogenic dissections caused by trauma from guide wires, catheters, or angioplasty balloons during angiographic procedures.
- Renal artery dissection can rarely occur as a result of trauma to the abdomen or flank.
- Chronic dissections are most frequently associated with fibromuscular dysplasia of the renal artery. Chronic renal artery dissection should be considered in the differential diagnosis of renovascular or difficult to treat hypertension.

## ■ Treatment

- Surgical revascularization may be beneficial to salvage renal function or to treat renovascular hypertension that persists despite antihypertensive therapy.
- In some patients, hypertension can be adequately controlled with medical therapy.
- Nephrectomy may be required when renal infarction has developed.

## ■ Pearl

*Because the most common symptom of acute arterial occlusion due to dissection is abdominal or flank pain, this diagnosis should be considered if more common conditions (such as gastroenteritis, pancreatitis, cholecystitis, nephrolithiasis and pyelonephritis) have been ruled out.*

References

"Nontraumatic Acute Occlusive Diseases of the Renal Arteries" and "Dissecting Aneurysms of the Renal Artery." In: Schrier RW, ed. Diseases of the Kidney & Urinary Tract. 8th ed. Philadelphia: Lippincott Williams & Wilkins; 2007:1788.

Smith BM et al: Renal artery dissection. Ann Surg 1984;200:134.

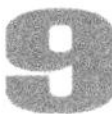

# Urinary Tract Infections

# Asymptomatic Bacteriuria

## ■ Essentials of Diagnosis

- Significant asymptomatic bacteriuria is defined as greater than 100 000 cfu of an organism in the urine on two successive urine cultures without symptoms.
- In a male one culture with more than 100 000 cfu of a bacterium is enough to diagnose asymptomatic bacteriuria.
- Found commonly in elderly females (25–50%) and residents of skilled nursing facilities (15–40%).
- Asymptomatic bacterial colonization rarely causes infection.
- Asymptomatic bacteriuria also commonly encountered in patients with an indwelling Foley catheter.
- *E coli, Staph saprophyticus,* group B *Streptococcus, Klebsiella* spp. are commonly isolated from pregnant females.
- Prenatal screening of pregnant patients for bacteriuria at 16 weeks.

## ■ Differential Diagnosis

- Early UTI.
- Catheter associated infection.
- Contamination of urine sample (check for squamous epithelial cells in sample).

## ■ Treatment

- Treatment recommended only in 3 settings: (1) pregnant patients, (2) Patients about to undergo urological surgery, (3) postrenal transplant patients (not in other transplants).
- Treatment of pregnant patients based on fact that they progress more quickly from asymptomatic bacteriuria to pyelonephritis and could more easily become septic.
- If recurrent UTIs, especially in pregnant patients, need to give postcoital prophylaxis.
- If not treated 30–40% of pregnant patients with asymptomatic bacteriuria will develop a symptomatic UTI.
- Amoxicillin/clavulanic acid, nitrofurantoin, cephalosporins.
- Avoid sulfonamides in the first and third trimesters of pregnancy.
- Avoid fluoroquinolones throughout pregnancy.

## ■ Pearl

*Postcoital prophylaxis indicated in women with frequent UTIs with TMP/SMX (80/400) daily or 3 times/week, TMP (100 mg) alone, or nitrofurantoin, 50 mg for 6 months to 1 year.*

Reference

Nicolle LE: Asymptomatic bacteriuria: Review and discussion of the IDSA guidelines. Int J Antimicrob Agents 2006;28 Suppl 1:S42.

## Funguria

### ■ Essentials of Diagnosis
- Common in patients with indwelling catheters and on broad spectrum antibiotics.
- Encountered most often in the ICU and in diabetic patients.
- Most commonly represents mere colonization.
- In cases of mere colonization removal of the catheter eradicates the colonized state in 40%.
- Diagnosis of an actual fungal urinary tract infection depends on the presence of other signs.
  - Fever.
  - Dysuria.
  - Signs of fungal sepsis (fever, bacteremia, etc).

### ■ Differential Diagnosis
- Fungal bladder infection.
- Fungal colonization.
- Systemic fungal illness.
- Contamination from fungal skin or vaginal infection.

### ■ Treatment
- Treatment of asymptomatic funguria is currently advised against by the IDSA.
- Fluconazole 200 mg can be given for 7–14 days and the catheter should be removed if the patient is symptomatic.
- Amphotericin 6 mg/kg/d and liposomal amphotericin 0.6 mg/kg/d (in renal failure) can be used to treat candidal pyelonephritis and fungemia.

### ■ Pearl
*A study of patients with positive candida urine cultures showed that contrary to what may be expected, patients who were treated for candiduria with antifungals were more likely to have subsequent positive urine cultures, and did not prevent the development of candidemia.*

Reference

Drew RH et al: Is it time to abandon the use of amphotericin B bladder irrigation? Clin Infect Dis 2005;40(10):1465.

# Urinary Tract Infections (UTIs)

## ■ Essentials of Diagnosis
- Most common in young females, typically caused by *E coli*.
- Clinical triad: dysuria, frequency, and urgency.
- History of dysuria and frequency is 96% sensitive, and warrants treatment.
- Urinalysis helpful in cases where history is less typical (95% sensitive, 70% specific).
- Urinalysis typically shows pyuria greater than 5 WBC/hpf.
- Dipstick + for leukocyte esterase is (70% sensitive, 85% specific).
- Cultures should be sent for patients with recurrent UTIs.
- Can progress to pyelonephritis and urosepsis if infection is not appropriately treated.
- Patients with indwelling catheters frequently have recurrent UTIs with resistant organisms.
- Diabetic patients are also at higher risk for resistant UTIs caused by different organisms such as *Klebsiella*.
- Imaging is indicated if anatomic abnormalities suspected.
- Urgent urological consult for emphysematous cystitis/ pyelonephritis, caused by gas forming organisms.
- Diabetics are at greater risk for infections by gas forming organisms.
- *Staphylococcus aureus* UTI can sometimes be due to hematogenous seeding of bladder.
- Nosocomial UTIs are often caused by highly resistant pathogens like *Pseudomonas, Klebsiella, Enterobacter, Enterococcus.*

## ■ Differential Diagnosis
- Cervicitis/urethritis due to *Neisseria gonorrhea/Chlamydia trachomatis.*
- Prostatitis in males/prostatic abscess.
- Ascending infection.
- Candidal or HSV vaginitis.

## ■ Treatment
- Uncomplicated UTI: 3 day course of TMP/SMX is first line.
- If suspect resistance to TMP/SMX, use a fluoroquinolone.
- 7 day course of a beta-lactam is another possibility.
- 14 day course of antibiotics for complicated UTIs.

## ■ Pearl
*Mycobacterium tuberculosis causes sterile pyuria and is an important cause of chronic UTIs in at risk populations.*

# 10

# Cystic Diseases of the Kidneys

# Acquired Cystic Kidney Disease

## ▪ Essentials of Diagnosis
- Four or more cysts in each kidney by ultrasonography or CT scan in patients with advanced chronic renal failure or in a uremic state.
- Absence of inherited cystic renal diseases.
- Strong association with renal cancer; tend to be bilateral, multifocal, and can be clear cell or papillary carcinomas.
- Usually asymptomatic; can cause flank pain infrequently, hematuria, or perinephric hematoma due to cyst hemorrhage or renal cancer.
- Normal- or small-sized kidneys.
- Cysts arise from cortex, walls are often calcified; papillary cystadenomas can be identified within cysts.

## ▪ Differential Diagnosis
- Autosomal dominant polycystic kidney disease.
- Autosomal recessive polycystic kidney disease.
- Multiple simple cysts.
- Glomerulocystic kidney disease.
- Tuberous sclerosis complex.
- von Hippel-Lindau disease.

## ▪ Treatment
- Bilateral nephrectomy indicated in cases of retroperitoneal hemorrhage, infection, and/or renal cancer >3 cm in diameter.

## ▪ Pearl
*Screening for renal cancer not indicated for all patients, unless patient has few comorbidities, good life expectancy and have been on dialysis for at least 3 years.*

Reference

Ikeda R et al: Proliferative activity of renal cell carcinoma associated with acquired cystic disease of the kidney: Comparison with typical renal cell carcinoma. Hum Pathol 2002;33(2):230.

## Autosomal Dominant Polycystic Kidney Disease (ADPKD)

- **Essentials of Diagnosis**
  - Two renal cysts unilaterally or bilaterally before age 30 years by renal ultrasound in patients with a family history of ADPKD.
  - Two cysts in each kidney between the ages of 30 and 59 years by renal ultrasound in patients with a family history of ADPKD.
  - Four or more cysts in each kidney after age 60 years or older by renal ultrasound in patients with a family history of ADPKD.
  - Renal manifestations include hypertension, flank pain, gross hematuria, urinary concentration defect, nephrolithiasis, urinary tract/cyst infections, or renal failure.
  - Extrarenal manifestations include polycystic liver disease, intracranial aneurysms, valvular heart disease, and renal cell carcinoma.

- **Differential Diagnosis**
  - Autosomal recessive polycystic kidney disease.
  - Acquired cystic kidney disease.
  - Multiple simple cysts.
  - Glomerulocystic kidney disease.
  - Tuberous sclerosis complex.
  - von Hippel-Lindau disease.

- **Treatment**
  - No definitive treatment to halt cystic disease progression or induce cyst regression.
  - Smoking cessation.
  - Treatment of hypertension with ACEI, ARBs, or $\beta$-blockers. Avoidance of high-dose diuretics because they may reduce renal blood flow.
  - Consider cyst decompression when conservative pain management strategies fail.
  - Prompt treatment of symptomatic urethritis or cystitis.

- **Pearl**

*Cysts arise from cortex and medulla, distinguishing ADPKD from other renal cystic diseases.*

Reference

Ong ACM, Harris PC: Molecular pathogenesis of ADPKD; the polycystic complex gets complex. Kidney Int 2005;67:1234.

# Autosomal Recessive Polycystic Kidney Disease

- ■ Essentials of Diagnosis
  - Recessive pattern of transmission; parental consanguinity.
  - Presentations for the neonatal period and infancy: oligohydramnios, Potter phenotype, pulmonary hypoplasia, specific facial characteristics (wide set eyes, beaked nose, low-lying ears), hypertension, urinary concentration defect, and large echogenic kidneys with poor corticomedullary differentiation.
  - Presentations for older children and adolescents: portal fibrosis, portal hypertension, increased hepatic echogenicity, hepatosplenomegaly, dilated intrahepatic ducts, and medullary sponge kidney and renal cysts.
  - Ascending cholangitis can occur at any age.
  - End stage renal failure can be associated with growth failure, anemia, and osteodystrophy.

- ■ Differential Diagnosis
  - Childhood-onset ADPKD.
  - Glomerulocystic kidney disease.
  - Nephronophthisis.
  - Meckel-Gruber syndrome, Bardet-Biedl syndrome, or asphyxiating thoracic dystrophy.

- ■ Treatment
  - Respiratory support for pulmonary insufficiency.
  - ACEI, ARBs, β-blockers for treatment of hypertension.
  - Splenectomy may be indicated in severe hypersplenism, leukocytopenia, and thrombocytopenia.
  - Dialysis and kidney transplantation in ESRD.
  - Prompt treatment of bacterial ascending cholangitis.
  - Serial monitoring for hepatosplenomegaly and varices. Primary prevention of variceal bleeding with β-blockers and/or banding or portosystemic shunting.
  - Liver transplant in severe hepatic complications.

- ■ Pearl

*With age, the size of the kidneys decrease, macroscopic cysts develop, and interstitial fibrosis is prominent, making the appearance difficult to distinguish from ADPKD.*

Reference

Bergmann C et al: PKHD1 mutations in autosomal recessive polycystic kidney disease (ARPKD). Hum Mutat 2004;23(5):453.

## Medullary Sponge Disease

- **Essentials of Diagnosis**
  - Precalyceal tubular ectasia with a pathognomonic "paint brush appearance" on excretory urogram.
  - Usually without a positive family history and with normal renal clearance.
  - May be associated with a variety of congenital abnormalities including congenital hemihypertrophy, Beckwith-Wiedemann syndrome, and Ehlers-Danlos syndrome.
  - May present with nephrolithiasis, recurrent urinary tract infections, and microhematuria.
  - Nephrolithiasis can lead to recurrent stone-induced obstructive uropathy.

- **Differential Diagnosis**
  - Autosomal dominant polycystic kidney disease.
  - Autosomal recessive polycystic kidney disease.
  - Acquired cystic kidney disease.
  - Glomerulocystic kidney disease.
  - Simple renal cysts.
  - Tuberous sclerosis complex.
  - von Hippel-Lindau disease.

- **Treatment**
  - Treatment of nephrolithiasis.
  - May need prolonged antibiotic therapy to treat urinary tract infections.

- **Pearl**

*Associated with tubular dilation, urinary stasis, hypercalciuria, and hypocitraturia, which are thought to contribute to stone formation.*

### Reference

Milliner DS et al: Urolithiasis. In: Avner ED et al(eds.) Pediatric Nephrology, ed 5. Lippincott, Williams & Wilkins; 2004: 1091-1112.

# Nephronophthisis & Medullary Cystic Disease

- ## Essentials of Diagnosis
  - Small kidneys with tubular atrophy and interstitial fibrosis.
  - Renal cysts located in the corticomedullary junction.
  - Can cause chronic renal failure with minimal and low-grade proteinuria.
  - Earliest symptom may be polyuria and polydipsia secondary to urinary concentration defect.
  - Nephronophthisis has autosomal recessive inheritance and is associated with retinitis pigmentosa.
  - Medullary cystic disease has autosomal dominant inheritance and is associated with hyperuricemia and gouty arthritis.

- ## Differential Diagnosis
  - Autosomal dominant polycystic kidney disease.
  - Autosomal recessive polycystic kidney disease.
  - Acquired cystic kidney disease.
  - Glomerulocystic kidney disease.
  - Simple renal cysts.
  - Tuberous sclerosis complex.
  - von Hippel-Lindau disease.

- ## Treatment
  - No specific treatment for renal dysfunction.
  - Treat hyperuricemia and gout with allopurinol.
  - Dialysis and transplant for cases progressing to end stage renal disease.

- ## Pearl

*Nephronophthisis has childhood or adolescent onset of end stage renal failure, whereas in medullary cystic disease renal failure occurs in adulthood.*

Reference

Bichet DG et al: The quest for the gene responsible for medullary cystic kidney disease type I. Kidney Int 2004;66(2):864.

# Renal Cysts, Simple

## ■ Essentials of Diagnosis
- Rare in individuals less than age 30 years.
- 1.7% of individuals at age 30–49, 11.5% at age 50–70, and 22–30% at age greater than 70 years have at least one renal cyst.
- Number and size of cysts increase with age.
- Conventional renal ultrasound underestimates the number of renal cysts compared to that of CT or MRI.
- In most cases are asymptomatic, however occasionally flank pain, cyst hemorrhage, hematuria, or cyst infection can occur.
- Commonly located in the cortex; usually present as round, smooth thin-walled with sharply defined margins without internal echoes.

## ■ Differential Diagnosis
- Autosomal dominant polycystic kidney disease.
- Autosomal recessive polycystic kidney disease.
- Acquired cystic kidney disease.
- Glomerulocystic kidney disease.
- Tuberous sclerosis complex.
- von Hippel-Lindau disease.

## ■ Treatment
- Only needed when pain, cyst hemorrhage, or cyst infection occurs.
- Cysts with internal echoes on ultrasound or those that show enhancement on CT with contrast require further diagnostic evaluation such as cyst aspiration and/or angiography.

## ■ Pearl
*Simple renal cysts have been reported to be associated with renin-mediated hypertension and erythropoietin-mediated erythrocytosis.*

Reference

Terada N et al: The natural history of simple renal cysts. J Urol 2002;167(1):21.

## Tuberous Sclerosis Complex

- ■ **Essentials of Diagnosis**
  - Major features include facial angiofibromas or forehead plaques, ungual fibromas, hypomelanotic macules, shagreen patch, retinal hamartomas, cortical tubers, subependymal nodules or giant cell astrocytomas, cardiac rhabdomyoma, and renal angiomyolipomas.
  - Minor features include dental enamel pits, hamartomatous rectal polyps, bone cysts, cerebral radial migration lines, nonrenal hamartomas, retinal acromic patch, multiple renal cysts, and "confetti" skin lesions.
  - Definitive diagnosis requires either two major features or one major feature plus two minor features.
  - Renal manifestations include angiomyolipomas, cysts, renal cell carcinomas, renal oncocytomas, FSGS with interstitial fibrosis, glomerular microhamartomas, and lymphangiomatous cysts.

- ■ **Differential Diagnosis**
  - Autosomal dominant polycystic kidney disease and autosomal recessive polycystic kidney disease.
  - Acquired cystic kidney disease.
  - Multiple simple cysts.
  - Glomerulocystic kidney disease.
  - von Hippel-Lindau disease.

- ■ **Treatment**
  - Semiannual or annual observation in slow growing or less than 4 cm angiomyolipomas.
  - Renal-sparing tumor resection versus nephrectomy in rapidly growing or more than 4 cm angiomyolipomas.
  - Arterial embolization of regional blood supply should be considered in highly vascular lesions.
  - Rapamycin is being tested in human trials as a potential pharmacologic agent to prevent tumor formation and growth.
  - In cases of ESRD on dialysis, bilateral nephrectomy indicated because of the risk of bleeding and cancer.

- ■ **Pearl**

*Imaging diagnosis of angiomyolipoma requires the identification of fat in the tumor, which shows as increased echogenicity on ultrasound or low attenuation on CT.*

Reference

Inoki K et al: Dysregulation of the TSC-mTOR pathway in human disease. Nat Genet 2005;1:19.

## Von Hippel-Lindau Disease

- **Essentials of Diagnosis**
  - Autosomal dominant inheritance.
  - In patients with a family history of von Hippel-Lindau (VHL) disease, a diagnosis is made if one of the following: cerebellar hemangioblastomas, retinal hemangioblastomas, renal cysts and renal cell carcinoma, and pheochromocytomas.
  - In patients without a family history of VHL disease, a diagnosis is made if one of the following: two or more retinal hemangio-blastomas, two or more cerebellar hemangioblastomas, or single hemangioblastoma plus visceral tumor.
  - Caused by a mutation in the VHL gene, a tumor suppressor gene.
  - Retinal hemangioblastomas can cause local hemorrhage, retinal detachment, and blindness.
  - Renal cell carcinomas are mainly clear cell type, have younger age of onset, have high risk of recurrence after resection, and are the leading cause of death.

- **Differential Diagnosis**
  - Autosomal dominant polycystic kidney disease.
  - Multiple simple cysts.
  - Tuberous sclerosis complex.

- **Treatment**
  - Surgical resection indicated for cerebellar hemangioblastomas.
  - Retinal hemangioblastomas treated with cryocoagulation or photocoagulation.
  - For renal cell carcinomas less than 3 cm, semiannual or annual follow-up with CT or MRI is recommended.
  - Tumor resection recommended for renal cell carcinomas greater than 3 cm given high risk of metastasis.
  - Humanized VEGF neutralizing antibody has been shown to delay the progression of metastatic renal cancers.

- **Pearl**

*Type 1 associated with truncating VHL mutations, and has low risk of pheochromocytomas, whereas type 2 associated with missense mutations, and has high risk of pheochromocytoma.*

Reference

Hines-Peralta A, Goldberg SN: Review of radiofrequency ablation for renal cell carcinoma. Clin Cancer Res 2004;10(18Pt2):6328S.

# 11

# Nephrolithiasis

# Cystinuria

## ■ Essentials of Diagnosis

- Autosomal, recessive disorder associated with defective transport of cystine, ornithine, lysine, and arginine in the renal tubular epithelium and GI tract. Types A and B cystinuria affect different genes, with Type A being more severe.
- Presents with cystine ureteral stones, which may lead to urinary tract infections and renal failure.
- Males more severely affected than females, though prevalence is equal among genders.
- Definitive diagnosis requires demonstration of hexagonal cystine crystals in the urine. Acidification of concentrated urine with acetic acid can precipitate crystals not visible on initial urine microscopy.
- The cyanide nitroprusside test may be performed on urine, resulting in a red/purple color if cystine is present in the urine.
- Cystine stones appear radiopaque on imaging.

## ■ Differential Diagnosis

- Patients with magnesium ammonium phosphate and calcium stones may also present concurrently with urinary tract infections, leading to a similar clinical picture.

## ■ Treatment

- Increasing fluid intake (up to 4 L/d) and reducing sodium in the diet may result in lower urinary cystine concentrations.
- Urinary alkalinization with potassium citrate may increase the solubility of cystine and decrease the risk of nephrolithiasis.
- D-penicillamine can bind to the cysteine molecules making up cystine to form a penicillamine-cystine complex that is much more soluble than cystine. Mercaptopropionylglycine works similarly.
- Kidney transplantation may be necessary if progression to ESRD occurs. A kidney from an unaffected donor will not form cystine stones.
- Extracorporeal shock wave lithotripsy is not helpful.

## ■ Pearl

*"Cys" sounds like "six." Cystine stones are hexagonal.*

Reference

Mattoo et al: Cystinuria. Semin Nephrol 2008;28:181.

# Hyperoxaluria

## ■ Essentials of Diagnosis
- Rare, autosomal recessive genetic disorder due to deficiency of an oxalate-metabolizing liver enzyme.
- Patients present with gross hematuria and renal colic during childhood.
- Excessive oxalate in the urinary tract combines with calcium to form calcium oxalate, resulting in nephrolithiasis and chronic interstitial nephritis.
- Majority of patients progressing to end stage renal disease by the second decade of life.
- Polarized light microscopy demonstrates birefringent positive crystals in the interstitial spaces and tubular lumens with surrounding inflammation and interstitial fibrosis.

## ■ Differential Diagnosis
- Other causes of chronic interstitial nephritis must be considered.

## ■ Treatment
- Maintaining a high urine flow may be beneficial to prevent nephrolithiasis.
- The recommended treatment for those with recurrent nephrolithiasis or end-stage renal disease is combined liver and kidney transplantation.
- Pyridoxine has been used with some success.

## ■ Pearl
*If renal transplant is performed without concurrent liver transplant, hyperoxaluria will persist, leading to recurrence of nephrolithiasis and renal failure.*

### Reference
Hoppe et al: The primary hyperoxalurias. Kidney Int 2009;75:1264.

## Hypocitraturia

- ### Essentials of Diagnosis
  - Low urine citrate (<450 mg/d in women, <350 mg/d in men).
  - Citrate is an inhibitor of calcium stones.
  - Low urinary citrate excretion may be a consequence of acidosis or potassium depletion or as an idiopathic disorder.

- ### Differential Diagnosis
  - Distal renal tubular acidosis.
  - Chronic diarrheal syndrome.
  - Thiazide diuretic use.

- ### Treatment
  - Increase urine volume.
  - Potassium citrate.

- ### Pearl
*Citrate inhibits stone formation due to its ability to chelate calcium, forming a soluble complex that prevents calcium binding to oxalate or phosphate.*

## Calcium Kidney Stones

- **Essentials of Diagnosis**
  - The most common type of kidney stone.
  - Can be calcium oxalate or calcium phosphate.
  - Radio-opaque on x-ray.
  - For calcium oxalate, the most important determinants of urinary saturation are the total daily calcium excretion and urine volume.
  - For calcium phosphate, urine pH is the critical determinant (solubility decreases as urine pH rises).

- **Differential Diagnosis**
  - Primary hyperparathyroidism.
  - Idiopathic hypercalciuria.
  - Granulomatous diseases.
  - Vitamin D excess.

- **Treatment**
  - Urine output greater than 2 L/d.
  - Low-sodium and low-protein diet.
  - Reduce dietary oxalate.
  - High dietary calcium intake.
  - Thiazide diuretic.
  - Potassium citrate.

- **Pearl**

*High dietary calcium intake decreases stone formation by binding oxalate in the gut, thus preventing absorption.*

Reference

Worcester EM, Coe FL: Nephrolithiasis. 2008 Jun;35(2):369, vii.

# Struvite Kidney Stones

- ■ Essentials of Diagnosis
  - Produced by urinary tract infection with urease-producing bacteria such as *Ureaplasma* and *Proteus.*
  - Large branched radiolucent stones to which bacteria adhere.
  - A mixture of magnesium ammonium phosphate and carbonate apatite.
  - Seen in patients who have urinary tract infections, neurogenic bladders, urinary diversion or in the presence of foreign material.

- ■ Differential Diagnosis
  - Calcium or other kidney stone.
  - Urinary tract infection.
  - Pyelonephritis.

- ■ Treatment
  - Treat with a combined medical-surgical approach.
  - Often too large for lithotripsy and must be removed by percutaneous lithotomy.
  - Antibiotics are ineffective in eradicating the infection when stone material is present.
  - Treatment requires both removal of all stone material and antibiotic therapy.
  - Acetohydroxamic acid (AHA) inhibits bacterial urease, and can prevent growth and formation of struvite stones, although use is limited by side effects.

- ■ Pearl

*Struvite crystals have a characteristic "coffin-lid" appearance on microscopy.*

Reference

Worcester EM, Coe FL: Nephrolithiasis. 2008 Jun;35(2):369, vii.

# Uric Acid Kidney Stones

- **Essentials of Diagnosis**
  - Occur due to low urine pH (<5.6) causing decreased solubility.
  - Represent 5–10% of all renal calculi in the United States.
  - Radiolucent on x-ray.
  - Stone formers are often obese or diabetic.

- **Differential Diagnosis**
  - Hyperuricosuria.
  - Lesch-Nyhan syndrome.
  - Fanconi syndrome.
  - Tumor lysis syndrome.

- **Treatment**
  - Potassium citrate to raise urine pH.
  - Decrease dietary protein intake.
  - High urine volume.

- **Pearl**

*In patients with uric acid stones, hyperuricemia and hyperuricosuria, consider inherited syndromes of uric acid overproduction, such as Lesch-Nyhan syndrome.*

### Reference

Worcester EM, Coe FL. Nephrolithiasis. In: Lerma EV et al. Current Diagnosis & Treatment Nephrology & Hypertension. McGraw Hill; 2009:345.

# 12

# Hypertension

## Adrenal Adenoma

- **Essentials of Diagnosis**
  - Also called aldosterone producing adenoma (APA).
  - The most important etiology of primary aldosteronism (40–70%) and idiopathic hyperaldosteronism or bilateral hyperplasia (30–60%).
  - Screening for primary aldosteronism is done by the measurement of serum aldosterone (ng/dL) and plasma renin activity (PRA) (ng/mL/h) and the expression of the results as the ratio.
  - HRCT or MRI can usually detect adrenal masses greater than 0.5 cm in diameter. Many adenomas are less than 0.5 cm and are therefore undetectable.
  - Three tests have been employed for confirmation of the diagnosis. The most common is the measurement of urinary aldosterone on the third day of a 200 mEq/d sodium diet. An excretion level more than 12 µg aldosterone/day is diagnostic. A second test is the measurement of serum aldosterone at the end of the infusion of 2 L of 0.9% sodium chloride over 4 hours. A value less than 7.5 ng/dL (or 5 ng/dL depending on the measuring technique) is normal.
  - Finally, less commonly used is the measurement of serum aldosterone after 3 days of a high-sodium diet plus the administration of fludrocortisone 0.1 mg four times a day. A value less than 5 ng/dL is normal.

- **Differential Diagnosis**
  - Primary hypertension.
  - Other causes of secondary hypertension.

- **Treatment**
  - The treatment of an aldosterone-producing adenoma is surgical excision using a laparoscopic technique if possible. Patients with idiopathic hyperaldosteronism should be treated medically with a mineralocorticoid receptor antagonist.

- **Pearl**

*Consider APA in patients with hypertension, hypokalemia, and serum aldosterone/plasma renin activity ratio greater than 30 and a serum aldosterone greater than 15 ng/dL.*

Reference

Funder JW et al: Case detection, diagnosis, and treatment of patients with primary aldosteronism: An endocrine society clinical practice guideline. J Clin Endocrinol Metab 2008; 93:3266.

## Coarctation of the Aorta

- **Essentials of Diagnosis**
  - Unexpected differences in BP in the extremities (eg, right > left arm, arms > legs).
  - Imaging study (typically echocardiogram) showing the site of coarctation.
  - More common in males (66–75%).
  - Differences in BP may be a clue to the location of the coarctation: If it is proximal to the left subclavian artery, SBP is typically higher in the right arm than the left arm. More commonly, the coarctation is more distal, and the SBP in the right leg is lower than that in the right arm.
  - The characteristic physical sign is a diminished or delayed left radial or right femoral pulse, in comparison to the right radial pulse. A loud systolic murmer is usually present, often with a thrill and occasionally heard in the back, accompanied by other murmurs (eg, bicuspid aortic valve, present in 50–80% of children). "Notching" (typically of the inferior posterior aspects) of the ribs (third through eighth) is characteristic, and the number and location of notched ribs may also provide information as to the location of the coarctation.
  - An echocardiogram can identify about 95% of coarctations through the first 8 cm of the descending aorta.
  - CT and MRI have also been used successfully.
  - Angiography may or may not be required.
  - Chest x-ray may show a 'Figure 3' sign (poststenotic dilation of the aorta).

- **Differential Diagnosis**
  - Takayasu arteritis and Moyamoya disease.
  - Other causes of secondary hypertension.
  - Aortic dissection.

- **Treatment**
  - An SBP gradient across the coarctation of more than 20 mm Hg generally requires surgical intervention.
  - Postoperative elevation in SBP is a predictor of long-term adverse outcomes (including death).
  - Aortoplasty has also been successfully used after an initial surgical repair. Hypertension recurs in about 25–33% of patients with repaired coarctation in long-term follow-up; exercise-induced hypertension is even more common (25–56%).

- **Pearl**

*Consider coarctation of the aorta when unexpected differences in BP in the extremities are seen.*

Reference

Prisant LM et al: Coarctation of the aorta: A secondary cause of hypertension. J Clin Hypertens 2004;6:347.

# Endocrine Hypertension

- ■ **Essentials of Diagnosis**
  *Primary Aldosteronism (See Adrenal Adenoma)*
  *11β-Hydroxylase Deficiency*
  - Second most common cause of congenital adrenal hyperplasia in some countries.
  - Autosomal recessive disorder.
  - Low renin, low aldosterone hypertension.
  - Hyperandrogenism.
  - Elevated secretion and levels of 11-deoxycortisol and deoxycorticosterone and decreased secretion of cortisol and aldosterone.

  *17α-Hydroxylase Deficiency*
  - Low renin, low aldosterone hypertension.
  - Rare genetic disorder, autosomal recessive, female phenotype in male patients.
  - Sexual infantilism in female patients.
  - Elevated secretion of deoxycorticosterone and corticosterone, no production of cortisol.

  *Apparent Mineralocorticoid Excess*
  - Low renin, low aldosterone hypertension, severe hypertension in very young patients.
  - Acquired as the result of overconsumption of licorice or its derivatives.
  - Abnormal ratio of the excretion of urinary free cortisol to urinary free cortisone or the ratio of the metabolites of cortisol and cortisone.

  *Liddle Syndrome*
  - Autosomal dominant disease.
  - Hypertension and hypokalemia, hyporeninemic hypoaldosteronism.
  - No response to mineralocorticoid receptor antagonists, good response to Na channel blockers.

  *Pseudohypoaldosteronism Type II or Gordon Syndrome*
  - Hypertension, hyperkalemia, metabolic acidosis, normal renal function.
  - Defects in the WNK1 or the WNK4 (without lysine kinases).

- ■ **Differential Diagnosis**
  - Other causes of secondary hypertension.
  - Primary or essential hypertension.
  - White coat hypertension.

- ■ **Treatment**
  - Surgical excision using a laparoscopic technique if possible for aldosterone-producing adenoma. Mineralocorticoid antagonist for patients with idiopathic hyperaldosteronism receptor antagonist.

Reference

Calhoun DA et al: Aldosterone excretion among subjects with resistant hypertension and symptoms of sleep apnea. Chest 2004;125:112.

## Essential Hypertension (Primary Hypertension)

- ■ **Essentials of Diagnosis**
  - BP ≥140/90 mm Hg in adults aged 18 years and older based on an average of ≥2 properly measured seated BP readings at each of two or more clinic visits.
  - Normal BP is a systolic BP (SBP) less than 120 mm Hg and diastolic BP (DBP) less than 80 mm Hg.
  - SBP 120–139 mm Hg or DBP 80–89 mm Hg is prehypertension.
  - Stage 1 hypertension: SBP 140–159 mm Hg or diastolic BP of 90–99 mm Hg.
  - Stage II hypertension: SBP ≥160 mm Hg or DBP ≥100 mm Hg.
  - Diagnosis should be interpreted in the context of the overall CV risk by evaluating other concomitant disorders and target-organ damage (TOD).
  - Affecting more than 29% of adult Americans, it is the most common reason for office visits to physicians in the United States.
  - People with a normal BP (<120/80 mm Hg) at 55 years of age have a 90% lifetime risk of developing hypertension.
  - A linear relationship exists between BP and risk of CV events.
  - All newly diagnosed patients should have evaluation of kidney function and assessment of CV risks as well as consideration for secondary hypertension.

- ■ **Differential Diagnosis**
  - Other causes of secondary hypertension, white coat hypertension and isolated systolic hypertension.

- ■ **Treatment**
  - Lifestyle modifications (weight loss, smoking cessation, moderation of alcohol intake, salt restriction, and increased dietary potassium intake).
  - Pharmacologic treatment.
    - o Low-dose thiazide-type diuretics should be used as initial therapy for most patients with hypertension either alone in stage I hypertension or in combination with other agents such as ACE-I, ARBs, calcium channel blockers, or β-blockers in stage II hypertension.
    - o ACE inhibitors or ARBs are indicated as agents of first choice in all patients with diabetes.
  - In patients with hypertension and diabetes or CKD, the recommended BP goal is ≤130/80 mm Hg.

- ■ **Pearl**

*Appropriate lifestyle modifications are strongly recommended for all patients with either prehypertension or hypertension.*

Reference

Chobanian AV et al: The Seventh Report of the Joint National Committee on the Detection, Evaluation, and Treatment of High Blood Pressure (JNC 7). JAMA 2003;289:2560.

# Fibromuscular Dysplasia (FMD)

## ■ Essentials of Diagnosis
- Typically affects young women (<50 years), accounts for 20–25% of renovascular hypertension. Patients generally do not develop renal insufficiency.
- The etiology of RAS is usually attributable to atherosclerosis (ASO) or fibromuscular disease (FMD).
- Medial fibroplasia will appear as a "string of beads" and is often located at the mid to distal portion of the renal artery.
- Hypokalemia may be a surrogate marker of hemodynamically significant renal artery occlusive disease.
- Captopril-stimulated plasma renin activity (PRA) testing may be preferable to PRA determination alone in the evaluation of the patient with renovascular hypertension (RVHT).

## ■ Imaging Studies for RVHT Diagnosis
- 1. Renal scintigraphy/renography; 2. Captopril scintigraphy/renography; 3. Renal angiography/arteriography; 4. Magnetic resonance angiography; 5. Spiral (helical) computed tomography scanning; 6. Duplex ultrasound scanning; 7. Renal resistive indices.

## ■ Differential Diagnosis
- Atherosclerotic renal artery stenosis.
- Other causes of secondary hypertension (endocrine hypertension, pheochromocytoma, adrenal adenoma, coarctation of the aorta, glucocorticoid remediable hypertension).
- Chronic essential hypertension.

## ■ Treatment
- Optimal control of hypertension and preservation of renal function, can be achieved either through medical therapy, percutaneous renal angioplasty (PTRA) with or without stenting, or renovascular bypass surgery.
- Optimal treatment of patients with RVHT remains an elusive goal because there are no randomized controlled trials comparing medical versus surgical versus renal angioplasty versus renal stents on BP control and/or the preservation of kidney function.

## ■ Pearl
*FMD is typically seen in younger female hypertensive patients compare to ASO which is generally seen in an older hypertensive population with concomitant diffuse ASO in other vascular beds (eg, coronary, carotids, and peripheral circulation).*

### Reference
Izzo JL, Black HR (eds): Hypertension Primer. 3rd ed. American Heart Association; 2003.

## Glucocorticoid Remediable Hypertension (GRA)

- ■ **Essentials of Diagnosis**
  - GRA, or familial hyperaldosteronism type I, a disorder with a chimeric gene formed from portions of the 11β-hydroxylase gene and the aldosterone synthase gene, resulting in ACTH stimulating aldosterone synthesis.
  - GRA is one of the causes of mineralocorticoid hypertension.
  - The specificity of the mineralocorticoid receptor for the natural and far more abundant glucocorticoid cortisol is similar to that of aldosterone.

  *11β-Hydroxylase Deficiency*
  - The second most common cause of congenital adrenal hyperplasia in some areas of the world.
  - Autosomal recessive disorder, low renin, low aldosterone hypertension, hyperandrogenism, elevated secretion and levels of 11-deoxycortisol and deoxycorticosterone and decreased secretion of cortisol and aldosterone.

- ■ **Differential diagnosis**
  - Other causes of mineralocorticoid hypertension.

  *Increased Mineralocorticoid Secretion*
  - Primary aldosteronism aldosterone-producing adenoma (APA), idiopathic hyperaldosteronism, adrenocortical carcinoma, congenital adrenal hyperplasia, 11-hydroxylase deficiency, 17-hydroxylase deficiency.

  *Increased Mineralocorticoid Action*
  - Apparent mineralocorticoid excess (congenital, licorice ingestion, ectopic corticotropin production, activating mutation of the mineralocorticoid receptor).

  *Increased Sodium Transport in Renal Epithelia*
  - Liddle syndrome, pseudohypoaldosteronism type II, or Gordon syndrome.

- ■ **Treatment**
  - Replacement of the cortisol deficit with hydrocortisone and the addition of mineralocorticoid receptor antagonists such as spironolactone or eplerenone.

- ■ **Pearl**

*The diagnosis is more easily suspected in young girls, as they present with virilization and hypertension. In boys and men, the diagnosis is suspected in young patients with low renin hypertension and sometimes pseudoprecocious puberty.*

Reference

New MI et al: Monogenic low renin hypertension. Trends Endocrinol Metab 2005;16:92.

# Isolated Systolic Hypertension

## ■ Essentials of Diagnosis
- Systolic hypertension is due to functional and structural changes in the aorta and large arteries.
- It is more difficult to treat than diastolic hypertension.
- Systolic BP increases linearly with age, while diastolic BP increases until about age 50 years and then declines.
- It is the predominant form in adults.
- It is not just "burned out" diastolic hypertension.
- It can arise de novo at any age, either preceding or without the presence of diastolic hypertension.
- Aging is not inexorably associated with systolic hypertension. In primitive or cloistered societies there is no relationship between age and BP.
- The risk associated with systolic BP is robust and log-linear irrespective of age.

## ■ Differential Diagnosis
- Pseudohypertension (spuriously high systolic BP readings due to abnormally stiff calcified peripheral arteries).
- Essential HTN.
- White coat HTN.

## ■ Treatment
- Lifestyle modifications (weight loss, smoking cessation, moderation of alcohol intake, salt restriction, and increased dietary potassium intake).
- Thiazide-based therapy in the systolic hypertension in the elderly program (SHEP) and calcium antagonist-based therapy in the systolic hypertension in Europe (Syst-EUR) study are clearly established.

## ■ Pearl
*Predominant clinical form of hypertension in middle-aged and elderly individuals.*

Reference

Effect of treating isolated systolic hypertension on the risk of developing various types and subtypes of stroke: The Systolic Hypertension in the Elderly Program (SHEP). 2000 Jul 26;284(4):465.

## Malignant Hypertension

- **Essential of Diagnosis**
  - It is a complication of hypertension characterized by very elevated blood pressure, and end-organ damage.
  - It is considered a hypertensive emergency.
  - Acute target-organ damage (eg, encephalopathy, myocardial infarction, unstable angina, pulmonary edema, eclampsia, stroke, head trauma, life-threatening arterial bleeding, or aortic dissection) require hospitalization and parenteral drug therapy.
  - Patients without acute target-organ damage usually do not require hospitalization, but they should receive immediate combination oral antihypertensive therapy. They should be carefully evaluated and monitored for hypertension-induced heart and kidney damage and for identifiable causes of hypertension.
  - Malignant hypertension with neurologic symptoms and advanced fundoscopic changes with papilledema should raise the possibility of RVHT.

- **Differential Diagnosis**
  *Identifiable Causes of Hypertension*
  - Sleep apnea.
  - Drug-induced or related causes.
  - Chronic kidney disease.
  - Primary aldosteronism.
  - Renovascular disease.
  - Chronic steroid therapy and Cushing syndrome.
  - Pheochromocytoma.
  - Coarctation of the aorta.
  - Thyroid or parathyroid disease.

- **Treatment**
  - Blood pressure goals are best achieved by a continuous infusion of a short-acting, titratable, parenteral antihypertensive agent along with constant, intensive patient monitoring.

- **Pearl**
  *Patients with end organ damage require hospitalization and parenteral drug therapy.*

Reference
Vaughan CJ et al: Hypertensive emergencies. Lancet 2000;356:411.

# Masked Hypertension

- **Essentials of Diagnosis**
  - Normotensive by clinic measurement and hypertensive by ambulatory measurement.
  - The underlying mechanisms are not well understood, but may include anxiety, a hyperactive alerting response, or a conditioned response.
  - 24-hour ambulatory monitoring is needed.
  - Studies showed masked HTN with similar risky condition to sustained hypertension.

- **Differential Diagnosis**
  - Essential HTN.
  - Secondary hypertension.

- **Treatment**
  - Life style modification with frequent BP monitoring.
  - Pharmacologic treatment for BP $\geq$140/90 mm Hg.

- **Pearl**

*It is logical to propose that there will be a significant number of people who are truly hypertensive but in whom the diagnosis is missed by clinic measurement. 24-hour ambulatory monitoring is precious.*

Reference

Thomas G et al: Masked hypertension. Hypertension 2002;40:795.

## Hypertension in Pregnancy

- **Essentials of Diagnosis**
  - Hypertension is the most common medical disorder of pregnancy and complicates a reported 6–10% of pregnancies.
  - There are four major hypertensive disorders in pregnancy:
  - *Chronic hypertension:* usually predates pregnancy or presents earlier than 20 weeks gestation. It is not associated with proteinuria and complicates approximately 3% of pregnancies.
    - o Those affected are at increased risk for superimposed preeclampsia, which complicates 25% of chronic hypertensive pregnancies.
  - *Preeclampsia:* pregnancy induced hypertension associated with proteinuria, that presents after 20 weeks gestation; in some cases, it can be diagnosed postpartum.
  - *Preeclampsia superimposed on chronic hypertension.*
  - *Gestational hypertension:* seen in 6% of pregnancies, it develops in the latter half of pregnancy and is not associated with features of preeclampsia (eg, proteinuria).

- **Differential Diagnosis**
  - Other causes of secondary hypertension.
  - Primary or essential hypertension.
  - White coat hypertension.

- **Treatment**
  - When maternal BP is more than 150/90–95 mm Hg, treatment should be instituted with BP generally targeted to 140/90 mm Hg.
  - The FDA classification designates most antihypertensives as category C (should be given only if potential benefits justify potential risks to the fetus).
  - Methyldopa remains the drug of choice; it has not been found to be teratogenic after a 40-year history of use.
  - Clonidine is another $\alpha_2$-adrenergic agonist.
  - Labetalol, a nonselective $\beta$-blocker with vascular $\alpha_1$-receptor blocking capabilities, is now widely used.
  - Hydralazine can be given PO, IV or IM; parenteral administration is useful for rapid control of severe hypertension.
  - ACEIs and ARBs are contraindicated in pregnancy.
  - The treatment for preeclampsia is delivery.

- **Pearl**

*There is little evidence that the treatment of mild to moderate hypertension in pregnancy reduces the incidence of superimposed preeclampsia.*

Reference

Milne F et al: The pre-eclampsia community guideline (PRECOG) BMJ 2005;330(7491):576.

# Renovascular Hypertension (RVHT)

## ■ Essentials of Diagnosis

- The most common cause of secondary hypertension in the United States.
- Diagnosis of RVHT can be made only if BP improves following intervention.
- The presence of anatomic renal artery stenosis (RAS) is not synonymous with RVHT.
- Progressive and occlusive renovascular disease may lead to impaired kidney function, termed ischemic nephropathy.

*Clinical Clues*
- Severe or refractory hypertension.
- Age of onset younger than 30 years or older than 55 years.
- Abrupt acceleration of stable hypertension.
- Severe hypertension in the setting of generalized atherosclerosis.
- Systolic–diastolic bruit in the epigastrium, flash pulmonary edema.
- Unexplained azotemia, ACE inhibitor- or ARB-induced renal dysfunction.
- Less common in African-Americans.
- More than 75% degree of RAS causes critical hemodynamic changes.
- PRA has been an insensitive method of screening with elevated levels present in only 50–80% of patients with RVHT.

*Imaging Studies for RVHT Diagnosis*
- 1. Renal scintigraphy/renography; 2. Captopril scintigraphy/renography; 3. Renal angiography/arteriography; 4. Magnetic resonance angiography; 5. Spiral (helical) computed tomography scanning; 6. Duplex ultrasound scanning; 7. Renal resistive indices.

## ■ Differential Diagnosis

- Other causes of secondary hypertension (endocrine hypertension, pheochromocytoma, adrenal adenoma, coarctation of the aorta, glucocorticoid remediable hypertension) and chronic essential hypertension.

## ■ Treatment (Medical and Surgical)

- For unilateral RAS, ACE inhibitors are preferred.
- Calcium channel blockers (CCBs) are effective in lowering the BP in patients with RVHT. They also maintain renal blood flow through vasodilation in the afferent arteriole.
- Surgical therapy: 1. Percutaneous renal artery intervention; 2. Percutaneous renal artery intervention for fibromuscular dysplasia; 3. Atherosclerotic renal artery stenosis; 4. Renal artery bypass surgery.

## ■ Pearl

*RVHT should be suspected in patients presenting with severe, sudden-onset hypertension prior to 30 years of age or after 55 years of age.*

## Secondary Hypertension

- **Essentials of Diagnosis**
  - Abrupt onset of hypertension.
  - Blood pressure $\geq$160/100 mm Hg.
  - Considerable target organ damage.
  - Positive result of a highly specific diagnostic test.
  - More difficult to control.
  - Particularly important in younger people. Diagnosing and treating secondary HTN will reduce the future burden of treatment and improve the quality of life.
  - The BP lowering response to specific antihypertensive drugs may offer important clues to the presence and type of secondary HTN. For example patients with renovascular HTN have an impressive response to ACE inhibitors and those with primary aldosteronism have better response to spironolactone.

- **Differential Diagnosis**
  - Essential HTN.
  - White coat HTN.

- **Treatment**
  - For some secondary causes of HTN specific and potential curative therapy is available.

- **Pearl**

*Abrupt onset of hypertension, usually blood pressure $\geq$160/10 mm Hg. More difficult to control, with considerable target-organ damage.*

Reference
Izzo JL, Black HR, eds. Hypertension Primer. 3rd ed. American Heart Association; 2003.

# White Coat Hypertension

- ■ **Essentials of Diagnosis**
  - Approximately 25% of those with hypertension have BP readings that are considerably higher in doctor's office or hospital than those measured at home, at work or by ABPM.
  - More common among elderly.
  - Higher risk for cardiovascular events and related mortality than normotensive, non-white coat hypertension patients.
  - Lower risk than those with primary hypertension.
  - 24-hour ambulatory blood pressure monitoring along with normal physical exam.

- ■ **Differential Diagnosis**
  - Essential HTN.
  - Secondary hypertension.

- ■ **Treatment**
  - Life style modification with frequent BP monitoring are recommended.

- ■ **Pearl**

*24-hour ambulatory blood pressure monitoring along with normal physical exam is needed and life style modification with frequent BP monitoring are recommended.*

References

Chobanian AV et al: The Seventh Report of the Joint National Committee on Prevention, Detection, Evaluation, and Treatment of High Blood Pressure: the JNC 7 report. JAMA 2003;289:2560.

Guidelines Committee: 2003 European Society of Hypertension—European Society of Cardiology guidelines for the management of arterial hypertension. J Hypertens 2003;21:1011.

# Pheochromocytoma

## Essentials of Diagnosis
- Tumors of neuroectodermal origin arising from chromaffin cells.
- Paroxysmal hypertension in 30–50%; sustained in 50%.
- Classic triad of headaches, palpitations, and diaphoresis.
- 90% benign, 10% malignant, 15% bilateral, 10% familial.
- 25% of patients with sporadic pheochromocytoma have a germ line mutation suggesting that they are founders.
- Biochemical diagnosis: measurement of urinary or plasma free metanephrines is more sensitive, and should precede localization efforts.
- Measurement of vanillylmandelic acid (VMA) is very insensitive.
- NIH proposed the use of plasma metanephrines as the most sensitive way of diagnosis; sensitivity of the test is very high, specificity is around 85%.
- Measurement of urinary fractionated metanephrines and catecholamines has a lower sensitivity (90%) but a higher specificity (98%).
- *Clonidine suppression test* is useful in equivocal cases. The test consists of administering clonidine 0.3 mg orally with plasma catecholamines and free metanephrines collected 3 hours later while patient is supine.
- A decrease of less than 40% for plasma metanephrines and less than 50% for plasma catecholamines is positive.
- Localization via CT scanning or MRI with T2-weighted images.

## Differential Diagnosis
- Clonidine or alcohol withdrawal, cerebrovascular events, migraines, and intracranial lesions.
- Drugs: ephedrine, cocaine, phencyclidine, and LSD.
- Panic attacks, hypoglycemic episodes, or hypertensive crises.

## Treatment
- The treatment of pheochromocytomas is primarily surgical.
- Patients are pretreated with an $\alpha$-blocker (phenoxybenzamine) and/or an $\alpha$-blocker (eg, prazosin, doxazosin, or terazosin) and a $\beta$-blocker (after the administration of an $\alpha$-blocker). A combined $\beta$-blocker and $\alpha$-blocker (labetalol) is particularly useful.

## Pearl
*The most dramatic presentation of a pheochromocytoma is an acute episode of severe hypertension, severe headache, palpitations, tachycardia, and diaphoresis.*

Reference
Pacak K et al: Biochemical diagnosis, localization and management of pheochromocytoma. J Intern Med 2005;257:60.

# Preeclampsia

- **Essentials of Diagnosis**
  - It develops in the latter half of pregnancy (after 20 wk) in 5–6% of all pregnant women, and is characterized by increased BP (>140/90 mm Hg) and new onset proteinuria (>0.3 g daily) in a woman who had normal BP before 20 weeks.
  - Worldwide, preeclampsia causes at least 63 000 maternal deaths yearly.
  - Eclampsia is the occurrence of seizures that cannot be attributed to other causes and complicates approximately 3% of preeclamptic women.
  - A severe variant of preeclampsia that features hemolysis, elevated liver enzymes, and low platelets (the HELLP syndrome) occurs in 1 in 1000 pregnancies.
  - Risk factors: nulliparity, multiple gestation, family history of pre-eclampsia (mother or sister), history of preeclampsia before 34 weeks in a previous pregnancy (40% recurrence), history of HELLP syndrome (50% risk of preeclampsia in subsequent pregnancy), obesity (body mass index more than 35), hydatidiform mole.
  - Age more than 40 years, underlying medical conditions, preexisting hypertension, preexisting renal disease, preexisting diabetes, presence of antiphospholipid antibodies.

- **Differential Diagnosis**
  - Secondary hypertension.
  - White coat hypertension.
  - Chronic essential hypertension.

- **Treatment**
  - Most cases of preeclampsia present close to term.
  - They are managed by obstetricians with an approach that includes bed rest, consideration of the use of antihypertensive.
  - Medications, and delivery of the fetus, followed by seizure prophylaxis with magnesium sulfate.
  - Lowering BP does not cure preeclampsia but may prolong the pregnancy, because uncontrolled hypertension is frequently an indication for delivery.

- **Pearl**

*If preeclampsia is diagnosed early, bed rest and close monitoring of maternal and fetal conditions may enable. Prolongation of pregnancy and improve maternal and fetal outcomes.*

Reference

Milne F et al: The pre-eclampsia community guideline (PRECOG): How to screen for and detect onset of pre-eclampsia in the community. BMJ 2005;330(7491):576.

# 13

# Selected Inherited Diseases of the Kidneys (Tubules)

## Alport Syndrome

- ■ Essentials of Diagnosis
  - Results from mutations in type IV collagen, which is the predominant constituent of basement membranes.
  - Can be inherited from either the x-linked (80%), autosomal recessive (15%), or autosomal dominant (5%) forms.
  - Persistent microscopic hematuria detected during childhood is a constant feature.
  - Associated with defects of basement membrane in cochlea leading to sensorineural hearing loss and eyes leading to anterior lenticonus and corneal abnormalities.
  - Presence of diffuse thickening of glomerular basement membrane with multilamellar splitting of lamina densa on electron microscopy is diagnostic.
  - Most patients reach end stage renal disease by the age of 40.

- ■ Differential Diagnosis
  - In children, persistent microscopic hematuria can occur in thin basement membrane nephropathy, IgA nephropathy, other forms of chronic glomerulonephritis, and hypercalciuria.
  - In adults, the differential diagnosis includes conditions mentioned above as well as urologic lesions, especially in individuals over 40 years of age.

- ■ Treatment
  - To date, no controlled therapeutic trials in patients with Alport syndrome have been conducted.
  - An uncontrolled study of a small number of males with x-linked Alport syndrome showed that cyclosporine reduced proteinuria and appeared to stabilize renal function.

- ■ Pearl

*Overt proteinuria develops in all affected males while proteinuria is a risk factor for development of end-stage renal disease in affected females.*

Reference

Kashtan CE: Familial hematuria due to type IV collagen mutations: Alport syndrome and thin basement membrane nephropathy. Curr Opin Pediatr 2004;16:177.

# Fabry Disease

## ■ Essentials of Diagnosis
- X-linked recessive lysosomal storage disease caused by deficient activity of α-galactosidase A (α-Gal A).
- Results in accumulation of globotriaosylceramide (GL-3) and deposition in vascular endothelium causes angiokeratomas, acroparesthesias, hypohidrosis, corneal changes, renal failure, cardiac and cerebrovascular disease, and early death.
- Females can clinically vary in symptoms from asymptomatic to as severe as classically affected males.
- Diagnosis made through mutation analysis by DNA sequencing of α-Gal A gene.

## ■ Differential Diagnosis
- Pain symptoms similar to other disorders such as rheumatoid arthritis, juvenile arthritis, lupus, rheumatic fever, multiple sclerosis, fibromyalgia, erythromelalgia, and "growing pains".
- Cutaneous lesions can also be seen in angiokeratoma of Fordyce/Mibelli/circumscriptum and other lysosomal storage diseases.

## ■ Treatment
- Enzyme replacement therapy with recombinant human α-Gal A recommended as early as possible.
- Avoid precipitating causes of pain (stress, exposure to sun or heat, changes in temperature, physical exertion, fever).
- Severe pain can be treated with medications such as phenytoin, carbamazepine, or gabapentin.
- Renal disease can be managed with low sodium, low protein diet, and presymptomatic treatment with ACE inhibitors or ARBs should be considered.
- Severe renal dysfunction may require hemodialysis and kidney transplant.

## ■ Pearl
*Disease progression is slow, and renal failure in classically affected males usually occurs between the ages of 35 and 45.*

### Reference
Desnick RJ et al: Fabry disease, an under-recognized multisystemic disorder: Expert recommendations for diagnosis, management, and enzyme replacement therapy. Ann Intern Med 2003;138:338.

# Proximal Renal Tubular Acidosis (RTA)

- ■ Essentials of Diagnosis
  - Caused by impaired proximal tubule reabsorption of filtered $HCO_3$, leading to urinary bicarbonate wasting.
  - Hyperchloremic normal anion gap metabolic acidosis.
  - Urine pH greater than 5.5 in acute phase or when patient is given bicarbonate supplementation.
  - Urine pH less than 5.5 in the chronic steady state.
  - Fractional excretion of $HCO_3$ is elevated (>20%) in acute phase or when patient is given bicarbonate supplementation.
  - Usually associated with low or normal serum potassium.
  - Common causes include: multiple myeloma, ifosfamide, amyloidosis, heavy metals, inherited disorders such as cystinosis, tyrosinemia, galactosemia and Wilson disease.

- ■ Differential Diagnosis
  - Carbonic anhydrase inhibitor use.
  - Distal renal tubular acidosis.
  - Diarrhea.
  - Ileal diversion.

- ■ Treatment
  - Sodium bicarbonate (such as sodium or potassium citrate) supplementation to maintain serum bicarbonate more than 20 mmol/L.
  - In children, should maintain serum bicarbonate more than 22 mmol/L.
  - Typically requires high dose of bicarbonate to replace urinary losses of bicarbonate (>5–10 mmol/kg/d).
  - Supplement potassium as needed.

- ■ Pearl

*Acquired proximal RTA in adults, especially associated with other proximal tubule reabsorptive defects such as glycosuria, phosphaturia, uricosuria, and aminoaciduria (Fanconi syndrome) must consider multiple myeloma.*

Reference

Rodriguez SJ: Renal tubular acidosis: The clinical entity. J Am Soc Nephrol 2002;13:2160.

# Thin Basement Membrane Nephropathy

- **Essentials of Diagnosis**
  - An inherited form of glomerular hematuria associated with defects in type IV collagen.
  - Patients have isolated microscopic hematuria, either persistent or intermittent.
  - Proteinuria and hypertension are rarely observed but when present may suggest progression of disease.

- **Differential Diagnosis**
  - In children, microscopic hematuria can occur in Alport syndrome, IgA nephropathy, other forms of chronic glomerulonephritis, and hypercalciuria.
  - In adults, the differential diagnosis includes conditions mentioned above as well as urologic lesions, especially in individuals over 40 years of age.

- **Treatment**
  - Most patients do not require any form of therapeutic intervention.
  - Treatment with an agent that targets the renin-angiotensin axis indicated in patients with proteinuria and/or hypertension.

- **Pearl**

*Family history usually negative for renal failure.*

Reference

Van Paassen P et al: Signs and symptoms of thin basement membrane nephropathy: A prospective regional study on primary glomerular disease—The Limburg Renal Registry. Kidney Int 2004;66:909.

# 14

# Complications of Dialysis

# Hemodialysis Access Thrombosis

## ■ Essentials of Diagnosis

- Hemodialysis access thrombosis (includes catheters, AV grafts, AV fistulas) is the leading cause of loss of vascular access.
- The most common cause of malfunction in HD catheters is intracatheter clotting.
- Synthetic AV graft thrombosis occurs more frequently than AV fistula, and is usually the result of a stenosis (90% cases). A stenosis in an AV graft is due to neointimal hyperplasia. Thrombosis will occur when a stenosis remains undetected.
- If access has a thrombosis, blood flow may be slow or stop completely. Absolute arterial negative pressure increases.
- In AV grafts/fistulas: in addition to the signs above, patient may also lose bruit and thrill.
- Evaluation for patency of access can be confirmed with palpitation, auscultation, U/S and injected contrast studies.

## ■ Differential Diagnosis

- Dislodgement of the hemodialysis needles, causing poor or no blood flow.
- Hemodialysis machine malfunction.
- Tip of HD catheter lodged against the vessel wall.

## ■ Treatment

- For intracatheter clotting, alteplase may reestablish patency. If unsuccessful, exchange catheter.
- Treat stenosis along the feeding artery/vein by angioplasty to prevent future thromboses.
- In thrombosis, percutaneous thrombectomy includes local installation of thrombolytics and/or mechanical declotting with snares.
- Surgical thrombectomy is also a viable option.
- Screening for stenosis and percutaneous angioplasty of the lesion are key to preventing thrombosis.

## ■ Pearl

*The diagnosis of hemodynamically significant stenosis can be confirmed by elevating the arm above the level of the heart: the prestenotic venous segment will be filled to full size with palpable high intravenous pressure, whereas the poststenotic vein will collapse. Prolong bleeding time after decannulation is also symptomatic of down-stream stenosis.*

References

Feehally J et al. Comprehensive Clinical Nephrology. 3rd ed. Mosby Elsevier, 2007.

Fine RN, Nissenson AR: Clinical Dialysis. 4th ed. Mosby Elsevier, 2005.

## Hemodialysis Cuffed Catheter-Related Bacteremia

- **Essentials of Diagnosis**
  - Catheter-related bacteremia is common.
  - Causative organisms: gram-positive cocci (*Staphylococcus aureus* most common), gram-negative rods, fungal organisms (rare).
  - Patients usually present with fevers and chills.
  - Some patients may have hemodynamic instability or the sepsis syndrome.
  - Two sets of blood cultures should be drawn from the catheter and peripherally prior to initiation of antibiotics.
  - There may be evidence of exit-site infection or tunnel infection on physical exam.
  - Patients with *S aureus* bacteremia should undergo transesophageal echocardiogram to evaluate for endocarditis.

- **Differential Diagnosis**
  - Exit-site cellulitis.
  - Endocarditis.
  - Pneumonia.
  - Diabetic foot infection.
  - Septic arthritis.
  - Pyelonephritis.

- **Treatment**
  - Loading doses of vancomycin and an aminoglycoside should be given empirically after blood cultures are obtained.
  - Once culture results are available, more specific antibiotic therapy should be initiated.
  - Standard of practice is to remove catheter and reinsert at new site after eradication of bacteremia.
  - If fevers or bacteremia persist after catheter removal, a search for metastatic infection should be undertaken.
  - If no evidence of metastatic infection, systemic antibiotics given for 3 weeks.
  - Catheter exchange over a guide-wire instead of new site may be attempted in those with limited access.
  - Catheter salvage with systemic antibiotics AND antibiotic locks in catheter ports, is possible in select patients.
  - Catheter salvage should not be attempted in patients with *S aureus* bacteremia or candidemia.

- **Pearl**

*Check MRI of back to evaluate for epidural abscess in patients with tunneled cuffed hemodialysis catheters and back pain.*

Reference

Fine RN, Nissenson AR: Clinical Dialysis. 4th ed. 2005.

# Peritoneal Dialysis Peritonitis

■ **Essentials of Diagnosis**
- Presents with cloudy peritoneal fluid and abdominal pain.
- Send effluent for: cell count with diff, culture, Gram stain.
- Criteria for peritonitis (2 out of 3 must be met): clinical signs of peritoneal irritation, WBC greater than $100/mm^3$ with at least 50% neutrophils, positive culture from dialysate.
- Causative organisms: gram-positive cocci (*S epidermidis* and *S aureus*) 60–70%, gram-negative (enterobacter, pseudomonas, acinetobacter)15–25%, fungi (2–3%).
- Peritonitis with multiple organisms or anaerobes: consider CT scan or surgical evaluation to rule out abdominal pathology.

■ **Differential Diagnosis**
- Appendicitis.
- Mesenteric vein thrombosis.
- Pancreatitis.
- Cholecystitis.
- Perforation of a gastric or duodenal ulcer.
- Ruptured or infected cysts.

■ **Treatment**
- Empirically treat with broad antibiotics to cover GPCs and GNRs. Modify treatment once culture results are known.
- Gram-positive: vancomycin or cephalosporin.
- Gram-negative: Third generation cephalosporin or aminoglycoside.
- Fungal: flucytosine PO or fluconazole PO or IP.
- Multiple organisms: add metronidazole and remove catheter.
- Indication for catheter removal: no response after 5 days of therapy, fungal peritonitis, replapsing peritonitis, peritonitis with severe exit site infection, infection with multiple enteric organisms.
- Treatment course: intraperitoneal (preferred) for 2 weeks.

■ **Pearl**

*Peritonitis is associated with increased fibrin clot production that can occlude the dialysis catheter. Add heparin to each bag of dialysate to prevent this problem.*

Reference
Vas SI: The Diagnosis of Peritonitis in Patients on Continuous Ambulatory Peritoneal Dialysis. Seminars in Dialysis 8;1995.

# 15

# Transplantation

## Acute Transplant Rejection

■ Essentials of Diagnosis
- Usually presents as asymptomatic increase in serum creatinine.
- Less commonly can present with fevers, chills, graft swelling and tenderness, oliguria, hypertension, myalgia, arthralgia, and volume expansion.
- Can be due to cell-mediated immunity (ACR) or antibody-mediated immunity (AMR).
- Usually occurs after the first week of transplantation.
- Diagnosis: allograft biopsy classified into the tubulointerstitial and vascular forms.
  - ○ Tubulointerstitial ACR: infiltration of lymphocytes and monocytes into the walls and lamina of tubules so-called "tubulitis".
  - ○ Vascular ACR: lymphocytes, monocytes and less often foam cells are found in the vascular intima and rarely extend into the muscularis.
- Risk factor: preexisting sensitization.
- Pathology: diffuse peritubular capillary staining for C4d.

■ Differential Diagnosis
- Prerenal AKI or acute tubular necrosis.
- Acute interstitial nephritis.
- Vascular problems: arterial occlusion, venous thrombosis.
- Urological problems: obstructive uropathy.
- Thrombotic microangiopathy.
- Viral or bacterial infections: BK virus, CMV.

■ Treatment
- High-dose steroids: first-line treatment and reverse about 75% of the first ACR.
- Antibody treatment: thymoglobulin OKT3 are usually used as the second-line treatment. May be used as first-line treatment in severe or vascular ACR.
- AMR is usually treated by IVIG, plasmapheresis, ribuximab, or bortezomib.
- High-dose IVIG (2 g/kg) or low-dose CMVIG combined with plasmapheresis are two commonly used treatment protocols for AMR.
- Rituximab has been used in severe cases with high level of donor-specific antibodies.
- Bortezomib has potential for treatment of both ACR and AMR.
- After successful treatment of ACR interstitial inflammatory infiltrate diminishes rapidly whereas edema, tubular inflammation, and tubular cell damage may persist for some time.

■ Pearl

*Allograft biopsy is the most definitive means of diagnosis.*

Reference

Nankivell BJ, Alexander SI: Rejection of the kidney allograft. N Engl J Med 2010;363:1451.

## BK Virus Nephropathy (BKVN)

- **Essentials of Diagnosis**
  - BK virus is a human virus with seroprevalence rate of 60–90% among adult population.
  - Following primary infection BK virus establishes a latency within GU tract and reactivates in the setting of immunosuppression.
  - BK viuria develops in 30–40% of renal transplant recipients, 10–20% develop BK viremia, and 2–5% develop BKNV.
  - In kidney transplant recipients is associated with a range of clinical syndromes including asymptomatic viuria with or without viremia, ureteral stenosis and obstruction, interstitial nephritis and BKVN.
  - BKVN commonly presents as a rise in serum creatinine 2–60 months after transplant.
  - The diagnosis is made by allograft biopsy showing BK inclusions in renal tubular and glomerular epithelial cells.
  - In the absence of classic histologic findings, distinguishing between BKN and acute rejection if challenging and requires additional ancillary studies such as immunohistochemistry, in situ hybridization, or electron microscopy.
  - The most widely used immunohistochemical stain is an antibody against the large T-antigen of Simian virus 40 (SV40), which identifies BK virus infections due to cross reaction.
  - Most of the centers screen for BKV in blood or urine: (a) every 3 months during the first 2 years posttransplant, (b) when allograft dysfunction is noted, and (c) with each allograft biopsy.

- **Differential Diagnosis**
  - Acute rejection.
  - ATN.
  - Drug toxicity.
  - CMV infection.

- **Treatment**
  - There is no well-defined protocol for the treatment of BKN.
  - The current treatment includes reduction or discontinuation of antimetabolites in conjunction with a judicious reduction in CNI therapy or other components the immunosuppressive regimen.
  - Switching from tacrolimus to cyclosporine or to sirolimus has resulted in resolution of BKN and viremia/viuria in some cases.
  - Antiviral therapy with low dose cidofovir or lefunomide has been used with variable response.

- **Pearl**

*The mainstay of treatment of BKVN is reduction in immunosuppression.*

**Reference**

Wiseman AC: Polyomavirus nephropathy: A current perspective and clinical considerations. Am J Kidney Dis 2009;54(1):131.

## Chronic Allograft Failure (CAF)

- **Essentials of Diagnosis**
  - CAF has replaced chronic allograft nephropathy (CAN) recently in the literature.
  - Etiologies can be divided to immune or nonimmune mediated factors.
  - Immune mediated include: prior episodes of acute rejection particularly after 6 months, number of HLA mismatches, presence of preformed antibodies at the time of transplantation, noncompliance to medications.
  - Nonimmune etiologies of CAF are: serum creatinine at the time of discharge, delayed graft function, donor age, poor organ, donor recipient size mismatch, vascular diseases in recipient, hypertension, smoking, infections, proteinuria after transplant and recurrent diseases.
  - CAF is second only to death with a functioning allograft function as the most common cause of late allograft failure.
  - Usually presents clinically as declining allograft function, often with proteinuria and hypertension.
  - Morphologically include but not limited to interstitial fibrosis and tubular atrophy (IFTA).
  - Chronic allograft disease index (CADI) is used in the biopsies to predict allograft prognosis.
  - If a cause of CAF is established, repeated biopsies may be unnecessary because repeated treatment may be unwise.

- **Differential Diagnosis**
  - Nephrosclerosis.
  - Chronic CNI toxicity.
  - Recurrence of primary disease.
  - Other etiologies for slow rise in creatinine.

- **Treatment**
  - Once IFTA develops it is irreversible, therefore every effort should be made to prevent CAF before it happens.
  - In the setting of failing graft CNI therapy should be reduced or even discontinued and nonnephrotoxic immunosuppressant should be continued or started.
  - Refer patients for dialysis access placement and retransplantation when other treatments are ineffective. Stop immunosuppressive medications in stepwise manner.

- **Pearl**

*CAF is the second most common cause of graft failure and is characterized histologically as interstitial fibrosis and tubular atrophy (IFTA).*

Reference

Nankivell BJ, Chapman JR: Chronic allograft nephropathy: Current concepts and future directions. Transplantation 2006;81(5):643.

## Immunosuppressive Medications: Mechanisms of Action

- See also Immunosuppressive Medications: Adverse Reactions.
- T cell activation required 3 signals, which can be used as a target for immunosuppression.
- Signal 1: is initiated by the binding of the antigen to antigen presenting cells (APC) to the TCR–CD3 complex. ATG, OKT3, calcineurin inhibitors (CNIs) target this signal.
- Signal 2: costimulatory signal provided by the engagement of CD80 and CD86 on APCs with CD28 on T cells leading to IL-2 release. Belatacept targets this signal.
- Signal 3: IL-2 bind to receptor and through mTOR lead to cell proliferation. Basiliximab and daclizumab, sirolimus and everolimus target this signal.
- OKT3 is a monoclonal antibody, which targets the CD3 receptor complex and cause endocytosis of T cell receptor (TCR) while ATG targets CD3, CD4, and CD8 on T cells.
- CNIs bind to calcineurin and inhibit its action as a phosphatase. This impairs the expression of several cytokines responsible for T-cell activation and proliferation.
- Basiliximab and daclizumab target IL-2 receptor (CD25) on activated T cells, hence complementing the effect of the CNIs.
- Azathioprine (AZA) and mycophenolic acid (MMF) inhibit gene replication and consequent T-cell activation.
- Induction therapy, if used, usually consist of high-dose steroid plus either anti-CD25 or ATG depending on center preferences and patient's immunological risk.
- The mTOR is a key regulatory kinase in the process of cell activation. Sirolimus and everolimus inhibit this kinase. They have been used in CNI-sparing or steroid withdrawal protocol in low risk patients.

## ■ Pearl

*Immunosuppression usually consists of a CNI (cyclosporine or tacrolimus), an antimetabolite (MMF or AZA) and prednisone with or without induction therapy.*

### Reference

Halloran PF: Immunosuppressive drugs for kidney transplantation. N Engl J Med 2004;351(26):2715.

# Immunosuppressive Medications: Adverse Reactions

- See also Immunosuppressive Medications: Mechanisms of Action.
- OKT3 can induce fevers, chills, rigors, headaches, pulmonary edema, and, less commonly, aseptic meningitis, acute respiratory distress syndrome (ARDS), and encephalopathy.
- ATG can induce fevers, chills, and arthralgia, serum-sickness syndrome and anaphylaxis.
- Cyclosporine can cause nephrotoxicity, hypertension, hyperlipidemia, gingival hyperplasia, posttransplant diabetes mellitus (PTDM), neurotoxicity, hirsutism, hyperkalemia, hypomagnesemia, and hyperuricemia and, less commonly, thrombotic microangiopathy.
- Tacrolimus has similar adverse reaction but with a lower incidence of hypertension, hyperlipidemia, hirsutism, gingival hyperplasia, and hyperuricemia, and a higher incidence of PTDM, neurotoxicity, gastrointestinal disturbances, and alopecia.
- Side effects of sirolimus and everolimus include hyperlipidemia, particularly hypertriglyceridemia, increased CNIs nephrotoxicity, mouth ulcers, thrombocytopenia, and impaired wound healing, proteinuria, peripheral edema, delayed recovery from ATN or delayed graft function, reduced testosterone concentration, and pulmonary toxicity.
- The most common adverse effects of MMF are GI symptoms plus leukopenia and anemia.

## ■ Pearl

*Immunosuppression usually consists of a CNI (cyclosporine or tacrolimus), an antimetabolite (MMF or AZA) and prednisone with or without induction therapy.*

### Reference

Halloran PF: Immunosuppressive drugs for kidney transplantation. N Engl J Med 2004;351(26):2715.

## Posttransplant Infections: General Principles

- **Essentials of Diagnosis**
  - Infections in transplant recipients follow a "timetable" pattern.
  - First month after transplantation: most frequently caused by bacteria and include surgical wounds, drains, Foley catheter, bacteremia from vascular access, pneumonia, and UTIs.
  - During months 1–6: Infections associated with postoperative complications or with enhanced immunosuppression can develop, persist, or recur.
  - Augmented immunosuppression is associated with an increased risk of infection with immunomodulating viruses such as CMV, HSV, VZV, EBV, HBV, and HCV.
  - Beyond 6 months following transplantation: the risk of infection in patients with good allograft function is similar to that of the general population, with community acquired respiratory viruses constituting their major infective agents.
  - Patient with multiple rejections who had repeated exposure to heavy immunosuppression are the most likely candidates for chronic viral infections and superinfection with opportunistic organisms such as *Pneumocystis jiroveci*, *Listeria monocytogenes*, *Nocardia* asteroides, and *Crytococcus neoformans*.
  - About 80% of infections in kidney transplant recipients are bacterial.
  - Infections in kidney transplant recipients can be difficult to diagnose because of alteration in the immune response.
  - It may be difficult to differentiate among and infection acquired from the allograft, from an exogenous source or from reactivation of latent disease in the recipient.

- **Differential Diagnosis**
  - Differential diagnosis of fever in kidney transplant recipient is broad and includes infection, graft rejection, drug allergy, and noninfectious systemic inflammatory response.

- **Treatment**
  - Antimicrobial therapy is given for prophylaxis to prevent from a common pathogen, empiric therapy when the infecting pathogen is not identified, and specific therapy is used to treat a diagnosed pathogen.

- **Pearl**

*The timing of an infectious episode after transplantation is critical.*

Reference

Fishman JA: Infection in renal transplant recipients. Semin Nephrol 2007;27(4):445.

## Posttransplant Infection: Important Microbial Etiologies

- **Essentials of Diagnosis**
  - CMV infection occurs primarily after the first month and continues to be a significant cause of morbidity for the first 6 months after organ transplantation.
  - Primary infection often results in more severe disease than reactivation or superinfection.
  - CMV can present as from asymptomatic seroconversion, mononucleosis-like syndrome with fever and leukopenia/thrombocytopenia to tissue-invasive disease.
  - *Pneumocystis jiroveci* pneumonia most often occurs 2–6 month after transplantation and present with fever, nonproductive cough, hypoxia or focal consolidations in CXR.
  - BAL with bronchial biopsy and staining is highly sensitive method for diagnosis of PCP.
  - *Candida* spp. are the most common fungal pathogens in the transplant recipients.

- **Differential Diagnosis**
  - Varies with type and time of infection.

- **Treatment**
  - Prophylactic TMP/SMZ can reduce the incidence of bacterial UTIs, PCP, *Listeria monocytogenes*, *Nocardia asteroides,* and *Toxiplasma gondii.*
  - Pentamedine, dapson or atovaquone are the second agents if TMP/SMZ cannot be used.
  - Nystatin or fluconazole is used for fungal prophylaxis.
  - Acyclovir, valganciclovir, ganciclovir is used for HSV and CMV prophylaxis.
  - Treatment of established CMV disease consists of 2–3 weeks of IV ganciclovir followed by a 2- to 4-month course of oral ganciclovir or valganciclovir.
  - In refractory cases addition of CMV hyperimmune globulin can be of therapeutic benefit.
  - Oral valganciclovir can also be used in treatment of CMV viremia.
  - Candidal UTIs require amphotericin B bladder washing or systemic antifungal therapy with fluconazole, amphotericin B, or caspofungin for fluconazole-resistant species.

- **Pearl**

*Prophylactic antibiotics and antiviral are important in posttransplant period and should be restarted after exposure to heavy immunosuppressives for treatment of infections.*

**Reference**

Fishman JA: Infection in renal transplant recipients. Semin Nephrol 2007; 27(4):445.

# Posttransplant Lymphoprolifrative Disorders (PTLD)

- **Essentials of Diagnosis**
  - The incidence of PTLD is 1–2%.
  - Usually seen during the first year posttransplant.
  - Non-Hodgkin lymphomas (Hodgkin disease, most common lymphoma in age-matched controls), are of B-cell origin and CD20+.
  - Notable association with Epstein-Barr virus (EBV) infection; seronegative recipients of an organ from a seropositive donor are at highest risk.
  - Extranodal involvement (CNS, liver, lungs, kidneys, intestines) is common.
  - The mortality rate is much greater with PTLD than with lymphomas in the general population.
  - The prolonged or repeated administration of lymphocytic-depleting antibody preparations is a significant risk factor for the development of PTLD.
  - PTLD may respond to withdrawal or drastic reduction of immunosuppressive therapy.
  - Viral infections, CMV infection, may serendipitously reduce EBV replication and the incidence of PTLD.
  - PTLD may be of donor origin in some patients.

- **Differential Diagnosis**
  - Severe rejection.
  - Viral infections.
  - Opportunistic infections.
  - Primary lymphoma.

- **Treatment**
  - Restoration of host immunity is probably the most important therapy for the control of lymphoid proliferation.
  - Patients with evidence of polyclonality are most likely to respond to reduction of immunosuppression.
  - For patients with monoclonal tumors, immunosuppression should be drastically reduced or discontinued altogether.
  - Results with conventional cytoxic therapy and radiotherapy have been disappointing.
  - Rituximab anti CD-20 antibody with or without sirolimus has been successful in some cases.
  - EBV-specific cytotoxic T-cell infusion (novel).
  - After successful treatment patients should not be transplanted for 2 years.

- **Pearl**

*Reduction or discontinuation of immunosuppression is the mainstay of treatment in PTLD.*

Reference

Evens AM et al: Post-transplantation lymphoproliferative disorders: Diagnosis, prognosis, and current approaches to therapy. Curr Oncol Rep 2010;12(6):383.

# Posttransplant Polycythemia

## ▪ Essentials of Diagnosis

- Erythrocytosis occurs in up to 20% of posttransplant patients.
- Common during the first 2 years posttransplantation.
- Rarely occurs in patients who had native nephrectomy therefore suggesting that it is the native kidneys, rather than the allograft, that is the cause.
- The cause of erythrocytosis appears to be related to defective feedback regulation of erythropoietin metabolism.
- Erythrocytosis is not related to erythropoietin levels.
- Elevated levels of insulin-like growth factor-1 (IGF-1).
- Peak incidence: between 8 and 24 months after successful engraftment.
- Risk factors: male gender, retention of native kidneys, smoking, transplant renal artery stenosis, a rejection-free course with a well-functioning renal graft, and adequate endogenous erythropoiesis prior to transplantation.
- 10–30% develop thromboembolic events, and 1–2% subsequently die of associated complications.

## ▪ Differential Diagnosis

- Renal artery stenosis, polycythemia vera, hypoxia related such as COPD, smoking, sleep apnea and living in high altitude, hemoglobinopathies, tumors (renal cell carcinoma, hepatoma, leiomyoma), cystic renal diseases.

## ▪ Treatment

- Hematocrit greater than 60% are associated with increased viscosity and thrombosis, and treatment should commence at a hematocrit greater than 55%.
- Low doses of ACEIs and ARBs are generally effective in reducing elevated hematocrit levels.
- Their mechanism of action may be related to the induction of apoptosis in erythroid precursors and to reduction of IGF-1 levels.
- Theophylline is an alternative to the use of ACEIs or ARBs.
- Phlebotomy may be required in resistant cases.

## ▪ Pearl

*Stenosis of the transplant renal artery may be contributory and should be considered in patients with the combination of hypertension, edema, allograft bruit, and erythrocytosis.*

Reference

Vlahakos DV et al: Posttransplant erythrocytosis. Kidney Int 2003;63(4):1187.

# Posttransplant Proteinuria

## ■ Essentials of Diagnosis
- Proteinuria is common in the early period posttransplantation.
- Prevalence: 15–30% at 1 year posttransplantation.
- Early, low-grade proteinuria has been shown to be correlated to donor age and cause of death, ischemia time, and acute rejection.
- Persistent proteinuria posttransplantation is defined as urine protein greater than 1–2 g/24 hours for more than 6 months.
- Persistent proteinuria posttransplantation has been attributed to chronic rejection, recurrent or de novo glomerulopathy, glomeru-lonephritis, diabetes mellitus, and chronic and acute rejection.
- Even a small amount of proteinuria is considered a risk factor for subsequent renal function decline and has been found to be associated with decreases in patient and graft survival.
- Proteinuria is associated with higher incidence of CV disease and mortality.
- Posttransplantation urine should be checked for protein at least once a year.
- Origin could be from native kidney and is hard to differentiate although proteinuria from native kidneys usually improves after transplantation.
- It can be a marker of recurrent or de novo glomerular diseases.

## ■ Differential Diagnosis
- Recurrence of de novo glomerulonephritis.
- Nephrosclerosis.
- Chronic allograft glomerulopathy.
- Medications (sirolimus, everolimus).

## ■ Treatment
- Reducing high levels of proteinuria with ACE-I or ARB may help to reduce levels of serum cholesterol and alleviate coagulation and other metabolic abnormalities associated with nephrotic-range proteinuria.
- Nephrectomy should be considered when native kidneys are the origin of proteinuria.
- Switching to different immunosuppressive medications should be considered in patients on mTOR inhibitors with proteinuria.

## ■ Pearl
*Posttransplant proteinuria is common and is associated with reduced graft and patient survival.*

Reference
Knoll GA: Proteinuria in kidney transplant recipients: Prevalence, prognosis, and evidence-based management. Am J Kidney Dis 2009;54(6):1131.

## Recurrent Disease

- **Essentials of Diagnosis**
  - More common in recipients of living related transplants.
  - FSGS is associated with high rate of recurrence and graft loss.
  - Risk factors (for FSGS recurrence): younger patients, rapid progression to ESRD, collapsing variant, and presence of mesangial hypertrophy in initial biopsy.
  - The strongest predictor of FSGS recurrence is the history of recurrence in previous transplant.
  - *MPGN type 2 (dense-deposit disease)* recurs in almost 100% of patients and often leads to graft failure therefore considered a contraindication for transplantation.
  - *MPGN type 1* recurs in about 20–30% of patients and leads to graft failure in about 50% of patients.
  - High rate of recurrence of the nondiarrheal form of TTP which lead to almost 50% graft loss.
  - Risk factors (for TTP recurrence): older age at onset, rapid progression of primary disease, living donors, and use of CNIs.
  - *Membranous nephropathy (MN)* recurs in 5–10% of recipients and leads graft loss in 25% of patients.
  - Histologic recurrence of IgA nephropathy is common. Allograft failure to IgA nephropathy is higher than once reported and may be as high as 25%.
  - *Henoch-Schönlein purpura* recurs in a high proportion of patients and leads to graft failure in about 25% of cases.
  - *Anti-GBM disease* recurs in 10–25% of patients but rarely causes graft failure.
  - *Diabetes* recurs histologically in 100% of patients. Graft failure in about 5–10% patients.
  - Patients with *SLE and ANCA-associated vasculitis* are at risk of recurrence.
  - Percentage of recurrence may increase in all diseases as graft failure caused by rejection declines.
  - Biopsy is needed for definite diagnosis.

- **Differential Diagnosis**
  - De novo disease in allograft.

- **Treatment**
  - Usually the same as treatment of primary disease.
  - Plasma exchange pre- and posttransplant can reduce the incidence of recurrent FSGS and TTP.

- **Pearl**

*Patients with primary FSGS should be assessed for proteinuria after transplant for early detection and treatment of recurrent disease.*

Reference

Ponticelli C, Glassock RJ: Posttransplant recurrence of primary glomerulonephritis. Clin J Am Soc Nephrol 2010;5(12):2363.

# 16

# Urinary Abnormalities

# Crystalluria

## ■ Essentials of Diagnosis
- Asymptomatic is more common than symptomatic crystalluria.
- Symptoms: dysuria, urinary frequency, hematuria, renal colic.
- Crystals in the urine may form stones (nephrolithiasis).
- *Acidic urine* forms uric acid, calcium oxalate, cystine, and other amorphous urate crystals.
- *Alkaline urine* forms magnesium ammonium phosphate (triple phosphate or struvite), calcium phosphate, calcium carbonate, ammonium biurate, and other amorphous phosphate crystals.
- Drug- or drug-metabolites can also form crystals.
- Certain crystals suggest specific diagnoses (see below).
- Crystal precipitation can cause tubular obstruction.

## ■ Differential Diagnosis
- Uric acid crystals (suggest gout).
- Calcium oxalate crystals (consider ethylene glycol ingestion, granulomatous conditions).
- Calcium phosphate crystals (associated with UTIs, RTA, HPT).
- Calcium carbonate crystals.
- Magnesium ammonium phosphate crystals (suggest the presence of urease-producing organisms such as *Proteus* or *Klebsiella*).
- Cystine crystals (suggest autosomal recessive cystinuria).
- Drug-induced (indinavir, acyclovir, triamterene, sulfadiazine, TMP-SMX).

## ■ Treatment
- Treat the underlying cause if possible (eg, discontinue crystal-precipitating agent, control uric acid levels in gout, control other risk factors for crystal formation).
- Aggressive hydration and pain control.
- Specific medications may be indicated (eg, thiazide diuretics for calcium crystals, allopurinol for uric acid crystals, potassium citrate to alkalinize urine).
- Surgical intervention may be necessary for obstruction.

## ■ Pearl
*Classic examples of distinctive crystal shapes include: calcium oxalate ("dumbbell-shaped" or "envelope-shaped" that appear bipyramidal when rotated), triple phosphate (rectangular with beveled ends described as "coffin lid-shaped"), uric acid (rhomboid or "needle-shaped"), and cystine (hexagonal) crystals.*

### Reference
Daudon M, Jungers P: Clinical value of crystalluria and quantitative morpho-constitutional analysis of urinary calcium. Nephron Physiol 2004;98:31.

# Hematuria

- **Essentials of Diagnosis**
  - Symptoms: dysuria, urinary frequency, urinary hesitancy, pain.
  - *Gross* (red/reddish-brown urine) or *microscopic* (>2 RBCs/hpf).
  - Hematuria can be inherited/familial (benign or nonbenign).
  - *Glomerular* or *nonglomerular* in origin.
  - Dysmorphic RBCs or casts on microscopy suggests glomerular origin prompting evaluation for GN, including possible biopsy.
  - Consider biopsy if proteinuria or nephrotic syndrome (proteinuria >3.5 g/1.73 m$^2$/d plus other clinical findings) is present or worsening renal function of unknown origin.
  - Increased risk of kidney, ureter, and bladder cancers with smoking or chronic analgesic use.
  - Consider postponing evaluation if menstruating or postpartum.

- **Differential Diagnosis**
  - Renal or genitourinary malignancy (eg, prostate, ureteral, bladder, urethral, others).
  - Obstruction (eg, nephrolithiasis, BPH, prostate or other malignancy, others).
  - Glomerulonephritis (eg, postinfectious, membranous, others).
  - Renal vasculitis (eg, Wegener, Churg-Strauss, MPA).
  - Hemoglobinuria (eg, hemolysis).
  - Myoglobinuria (eg, myositis, rhabdomyolysis).
  - Benign (eg, benign familial hematuria, thin basement membrane disease, others) and non-benign familial causes (eg, PCKD, Alport syndrome, IgAN, sickle cell nephropathy, others).
  - Trauma or exercise-induced hematuria, UTIs.

- **Treatment**
  - Treat the underlying cause if possible and maintain adequate volume status, tissue/organ perfusion, electrolyte balance, and urine output.
  - Treatment may range from no treatment (eg, benign familial causes) to immunosuppression (eg, GN, renal vasculitis).
  - Manage BPH conservatively (medication) unless surgical intervention is necessary (eg, TURP).
  - Consider urologic evaluation for persistent or obstructive nephrolithiasis and antibiotics for UTIs.

- **Pearl**

*Gross or microscopic hematuria in patients ≥50 years old should prompt evaluation to rule-out genitourinary tract malignancy.*

Reference

Kincaid-Smith P, Fairley K: The investigation of hematuria. Semin Nephrol 2005;25:127.

# Hemoglobinuria

## ■ Essentials of Diagnosis
- Symptoms: dysuria, urinary frequency, pallor, purpura, pain.
- Urine color can range from pink to dark red.
- Occurs when RBC breakdown exceeds the capacity of binding-proteins (eg, haptoglobin) to bind free hemoglobin; whereas bound hemoglobin is too large for filtration, free hemoglobin is filtered, reabsorbed, and degraded by tubular epithelial cells.
- Red sediment following urine centrifugation suggests hematuria, whereas red supernatant that is heme-positive by dipstick suggests hemoglobinuria (clear in myoglobinuria).
- Absence of RBCs or casts or presence of dysmorphic RBCs (eg, schistocytes, spherocytes) on microscopy suggests hemolysis.
- *Intrinsic* hemolytic factors include abnormalities of the cyto-skeleton or cell membrane (eg, hereditary spherocytosis, paroxysmal nocturnal hemoglobinuria), metabolism (eg, G6PD deficiency, scurvy), and hemoglobin (eg, sickle cell disease).
- *Extrinsic* hemolytic factors include immune-mediated (eg, auto-immune hemolytic anemia, transfusion reactions), osmotic stress (ie, hypo- or hypertonic solutions), mechanical stress (eg, prosthetic heart valves, cardiac assist devices), micro-angiopathies (eg, DIC, TTP-HUS), drugs (see below), venoms (eg, snakes, spiders), chemicals (eg, arsenic, benzene), infections (eg, malaria, typhoid fever), and hypophosphatemia.
- Drugs associated with hemoglobinuria include penicillins, cefotetan, rifampin, minocycline, ribavirin, NSAIDs, IVIG, some chemotherapeutic agents, quinine, and other oxidants.
- Additional hemolysis studies include serum LDH ($\uparrow$) haptoglobin ($\downarrow$), and free hemoglobin ($\uparrow$).
- AKI, hyperkalemia, and metabolic acidosis may occur if severe.

## ■ Differential Diagnosis
- Gross or microscopic hematuria (glomerular or nonglomerular).
- Myoglobinuria (eg, myositis, rhabdomyolysis).

## ■ Treatment
- Treat the underlying cause of hemoglobinuria if possible (usually hemolysis) and maintain adequate volume status, tissue/organ perfusion, electrolyte balance, and urine output.

## ■ Pearl
*Avoid unnecessary transfusions. Steroids are indicated for immune-mediated hemolysis. Plasmapheresis may become necessary.*

Reference

Brodsky RA: Advances in the diagnosis and therapy of paroxysmal nocturnal hemoglobinuria. Blood Rev 2008;22:65.

# Isosthenuria & Hyposthenuria

- **Essentials of Diagnosis**
  - May be an incidental finding on routine urinalysis.
  - *Isosthenuria* occurs when urine specific gravity is equal to that of protein-free plasma (ie, urine osmolality = plasma osmolality) and remains constant around 1.010 irrespective of fluid intake or changes in the osmotic pressure of blood.
  - In *isosthenuria,* the renal tubules lose the ability to concentrate or dilute urine, therefore the glomerular filtrate remains unchanged despite the need to conserve or excrete free water based on volume or hydration status.
  - *Isosthenuria* may be observed in advanced CKD, but can also occur with AKI.
  - *Hyposthenuria* occurs when urine specific gravity is not equal to that of protein-free plasma, but is relatively low and remains persistently low irrespective of fluid intake or changes in the osmotic pressure of blood.
  - In *hyposthenuria,* the renal tubules can still concentrate and dilute urine, but within a limited range near plasma osmolality, therefore the glomerular filtrate is not altered enough to meet the need to conserve or excrete free water based on volume or hydration status.
  - *Hyposthenuria* is associated with certain hypokalemic salt-losing tubulopathies, sickle cell nephropathy, and diabetes insipidus.

- **Treatment**
  - Treat the underlying cause if possible (eg, therapies that slow the progression of CKD, therapy to treat diabetes insipidus, no specific treatment for sickle cell trait).
  - Appropriate management of volume and/or hydration status.
  - Late-stage CKD patients may soon require renal replacement therapy.

- **Pearl**

*Consider screening African American patients with persistent hyposthenuria for sickle cell trait, especially those with a family history of sickle cell trait or disease.*

Reference

Peters M et al: Clinical presentation of genetically defined patients with hypokalemic salt-losing tubulopathies. Am J Med 2002;112:183.

# Microalbuminuria

## ■ Essentials of Diagnosis
- Symptoms: urinary frequency, foamy urine, or asymptomatic.
- Defined as urinary albumin excretion of 30–300 mg/d or 30–300 mg/g creatinine.
- Quantify albumin by 24-h urine collection (preferred) or calculate the albumin-to-creatinine ratio (convenient) which correlates well with 24-hour urine albumin.
- Standard dipsticks do not detect microalbuminuria; albumin dipsticks (semi-quantitative) are available for screening, but laboratory testing (quantitative) is required when positive.
- The earliest marker of diabetic nephropathy (most common cause of ESRD), identifies patients at risk for progressive CKD and development of overt nephropathy, and an independent risk factor for cardiovascular events in diabetics and nondiabetics.
- Defines diabetic nephropathy stage 2 (of 5), typically occurring 5–15 years after diagnosis with diabetes.
- Persistent microalbuminuria increases the risk of development of overt proteinuria/nephropathy, progressive CKD.
- Reflects a state of endothelial dysfunction associated with renal microvascular disease; usually implies a defect in glomerular permeability allowing increased filtration of albumin.

## ■ Differential Diagnosis
- Overt proteinuria (>300 mg/d or 300 mg/g creatinine).
- Orthostatic, postural, or exercise-induced microalbuminuria.

## ■ Treatment
- Maintain blood pressure ≤130/80 mm Hg (preferably by blockade of the renin-angiotensin-aldosterone system) and control diabetes.
- ACE inhibitors and ARBs reduce intraglomerular capillary hydrostatic pressure, microalbuminuria, progression to overt diabetic nephropathy, blood pressure, and cardiovascular risk.
- Titrate ACE inhibitor or ARB to maximum dose for maximum benefit; however, there is insufficient evidence to recommend combination therapy even for persistent microalbuminuria.

## ■ Pearl
*Patients with diabetes (and ideally hypertension) should be screened annually for microalbuminuria and treated aggressively when present to reduce the risk of developing progressive renal failure, overt nephropathy, and cardiovascular mortality.*

Reference
Chugh A, Bakris GL: Microalbuminuria: what is it? Why is it important? What should be done about it? An update. J Clin Hypertens 2007;9:196.

# Myoglobinuria

## ■ Essentials of Diagnosis

- Symptoms: dysuria, urinary frequency, myalgia, weakness, pain.
- Typically occurs due to inflammation or lysis of myocytes (eg, myositis, rhabdomyolysis).
- Unlike hemoglobin, myoglobin does not have a specific binding protein and therefore does not accumulate in plasma; plasma is clear, but urine can range from pink to dark red urine.
- Absence of RBCs or RBC casts or the presence of dysmorphic RBCs (eg, schistocytes, spherocytes, others) on microscopy suggests hemolysis, not myositis or rhabdomyolysis.
- Myositis can occur due to drug-reactions (eg, statins, others) or infections (eg, viral, others).
- Rhabdomyolysis can occur due to trauma (eg, crush injuries, compartment syndrome), excessive muscle activity (eg, seizures), drugs and toxins, and prolonged immobilization.
- Additional myositis or rhabdomyolysis studies include serum CPK ($\uparrow$), aldolase ($\uparrow$), glutamic-oxaloacetic transaminase ($\uparrow$), urine myoglobin ($\uparrow$), and urine pH ($\downarrow$).
- AKI, hyperkalemia, and metabolic acidosis may occur if severe.

## ■ Differential Diagnosis

- Gross or microscopic hematuria (glomerular or non-glomerular).
- Hemoglobinuria (eg, hemolysis).

## ■ Treatment

- Treat the underlying cause of myoglobinuria if possible (ie, myositis, rhabdomyolysis) and maintain adequate volume status, tissue/organ perfusion, electrolyte balance, and urine output.
- Treat the underlying cause of myositis (eg, discontinue statins, viral infections) or rhabdomyolysis (eg, crush injuries, compartment syndrome).
- Treatment may range from no treatment (eg, mild or transient cases) to fasciotomy or amputation (eg, severe or traumatic cases) and may include urine alkalization (eg, $NaHCO_3$) to prevent myoglobin precipitation and tubular obstruction.
- Steroids are sometimes used for myositis (no proven benefit).

## ■ Pearl

*Rhabdomyolysis due to trauma or postsurgery should prompt evaluation of extremities for compartment syndrome, a medical emergency that may require fasciotomy to preserve limb viability.*

### Reference

Bagley WH et al: Rhabdomyolysis. Intern Emerg Med 2007;2:210.

# Proteinuria

- **Essentials of Diagnosis**
  - Symptoms: urinary frequency, foamy urine, edema.
  - Defined as urinary protein excretion of more than 300 mg/d or 300 mg/g creatinine (normal urinary protein excretion is ≤150 mg/d).
  - Quantify protein by 24-h urine collection (preferred) or calculate the protein-to-creatinine ratio (convenient) which correlates well with 24-h urine protein.
  - Urine dipstick detects albumin (not LMW proteins) when levels are greater than 300–500 mg/d (ie, does not detect microalbuminuria).
  - LMW proteins: myeloma light chain, Bence-Jones protein.
  - Usually implies a defect in glomerular permeability allowing increased capillary filtration of protein, but is commonly classified as *glomerular, tubular,* or *overflow proteinuria.*
  - *Glomerular proteinuria* is usually caused by increased filtration of albumin across glomerular capillaries due to glomerular disorders (eg, diabetic nephropathy, others).
  - *Tubular proteinuria* is usually caused by tubulointerstitial disorders that impair proximal tubular protein reabsorption.
  - *Overflow proteinuria* is usually caused by overproduction of protein that, when filtered, exceeds tubular reabsorption capacity (eg, myeloma light chain, Bence-Jones protein).

- **Differential Diagnosis**
  - Microalbuminuria (30–300 mg/d or 300 mg/g creatinine).
  - Nephrotic syndrome (>3.5 g/1.73 $m^2$/d plus other indicators).
  - Myeloma light chain or Bence-Jones proteinuria (LMW proteins).
  - Hemoglobinuria or myoglobinuria.
  - Amyloid proteinuria.
  - Orthostatic, postural, or exercise-induced proteinuria.

- **Treatment**
  - Treat the underlying cause if possible (eg, control glucose and blood pressure for diabetic nephropathy, immunosuppression for GN, no specific treatment for thin BM disease).
  - ACE inhibitors and ARBs reduce proteinuria by decreasing intra-glomerular capillary hydrostatic pressure.

- **Pearl**

*A 24-h urine protein greater than 3.5 g/1.73 $m^2$ should prompt consideration of renal biopsy, especially when associated with hypoalbuminemia (<3 g/dL), edema, hyperlipidemia, and lipiduria (ie, nephrotic syndrome) or in the absence of an obvious cause.*

Reference

Maione A et al: Proteinuria and clinical outcomes in hypertensive patients. Am J Hypertens 2009;22:1137.

# Red Urine

## ■ Essentials of Diagnosis
- Symptoms: dysuria, urinary frequency, urinary hesitancy, pain.
- Due to RBCs, hemoglobin, myoglobin, other substances.
- Red sediment following urine centrifugation suggests hematuria, whereas red supernatant that is heme-positive by dipstick suggests hemoglobinuria (clear in myoglobinuria).
- Hematuria (RBCs) can be glomerular or nonglomerular; dysmorphic RBCs or RBC casts on microscopy suggests glomerular origin prompting evaluation for GN, including possible biopsy.
- Hemoglobinuria without RBCs or RBC casts or with schistocytes on microscopy suggests hemolysis; additional studies include serum LDH ($\uparrow$) haptoglobin ($\downarrow$), and free hemoglobin ($\uparrow$).
- Myoglobinuria without RBCs, RBC casts, or schistocytes on microscopy suggests myositis or rhabdomyolysis; additional studies include serum CPK ($\uparrow$), aldolase ($\uparrow$), glutamic-oxaloacetic transaminase ($\uparrow$), urine myoglobin ($\uparrow$), and urine pH ($\downarrow$).

## ■ Differential Diagnosis
- Gross hematuria (glomerular or nonglomerular in origin).
- Hemoglobinuria (eg, hemolysis).
- Myoglobinuria (eg, myositis or rhabdomyolysis).
- Acute tubular necrosis (tea or cola-colored urine).
- Medications (rifampin, phenothiazine, phenazopyridine).
- Other substances (red beets in certain individuals).

## ■ Treatment
- Treat the underlying cause of hematuria, hemoglobinuria, or myoglobinuria and maintain adequate volume status, tissue/organ perfusion, electrolyte balance, and urine output.
- Hematuria treatment may range from no treatment (eg, benign familial causes) to immunosuppression (eg, GN, vasculitis).
- Hemolysis treatment may range from no treatment (eg, mild or transient cases) to splenectomy (eg, persistent hemolysis).
- Rhabdomyolysis treatment may range from no treatment (eg, mild or transient cases) to urine alkalization (eg, $NaHCO_3$) to prevent myoglobin precipitation and tubular obstruction.

## ■ Pearl
*Malignancies, nephrolithiasis, and GN are common causes of gross hematuria; hemolysis is the most common cause of hemoglobinuria; statins and viral illnesses are common causes are myositis.*

Reference
Patel HP: The abnormal urinalysis. Pediatr Clin North Am 2006;53:325.

# Index

Made in the USA
Monee, IL
15 May 2026